煤工尘肺病理学图谱

Pathology Atlas of Coal Workers' Pneumoconiosis

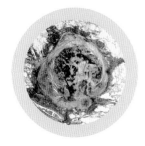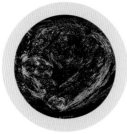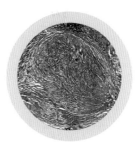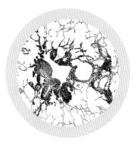

主 编　杨　方　孙　影　刘和亮

编 者　杨　方　孙　影　刘和亮
　　　　宋旭东　徐　洪　魏中秋

人民卫生出版社
·北京·

图书在版编目（CIP）数据

煤工尘肺病理学图谱 / 杨方，孙影，刘和亮主编
. —北京：人民卫生出版社，2020.12
ISBN 978-7-117-31073-4

Ⅰ. ①煤… Ⅱ. ①杨… ②孙… ③刘… Ⅲ. ①煤尘 –
尘肺 – 病理学 – 诊断学 – 图谱 Ⅳ. ①R598.204–64

中国版本图书馆 CIP 数据核字（2021）第 007848 号

| 人卫智网 | www.ipmph.com | 医学教育、学术、考试、健康，购书智慧智能综合服务平台 |
| 人卫官网 | www.pmph.com | 人卫官方资讯发布平台 |

煤工尘肺病理学图谱
Meigong Chenfei Binglixue Tupu

主　　编：杨　方　孙　影　刘和亮
出版发行：人民卫生出版社（中继线 010-59780011）
地　　址：北京市朝阳区潘家园南里 19 号
邮　　编：100021
E - mail：pmph @ pmph.com
购书热线：010-59787592　010-59787584　010-65264830
印　　刷：三河市宏达印刷有限公司（胜利）
经　　销：新华书店
开　　本：787 × 1092　1/16　印张：14
字　　数：341 千字
版　　次：2020 年 12 月第 1 版
印　　次：2021 年 2 月第 1 次印刷
标准书号：ISBN 978-7-117-31073-4
定　　价：95.00 元

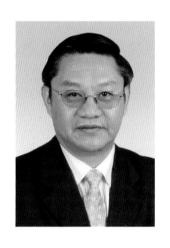

杨 方

华北理工大学教授／主任医师，博士生导师。河北省第十一届政协常委，唐山市第十届、第十一届政协副主席，民进唐山市委第六届、第七届主任委员。全国优秀教师，河北省省管优秀专家，河北省有突出贡献中青年专家，中国侨界杰出人物提名奖和贡献奖。曾任河北省医学会病理学分会副主任委员，河北省生理科学会副理事长，唐山市医学会病理学分会主任委员。发表论文 260 余篇（SCI 收录 60 余篇），主编著作 2 部，参编著作 1 部。主持与完成国家自然科学基金项目 3 项，国家 973 课题（协作单位负责人）1 项。省（部）、市（厅）级科研项目 10 余项。获河北省科技进步二等奖 2 项、三等奖 1 项，能源部、原卫生部科技进步三等奖各 1 项，中国煤炭工业科学技术三等奖 1 项，河北省教学成果三等奖 1 项。

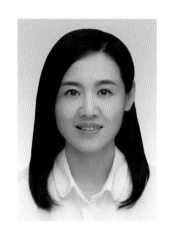

孙 影

华北理工大学教授／副主任医师，硕士生导师。华北理工大学基础医学院副院长／病理学系主任。中华医学会病理学分会心血管疾病学组委员，中华医学会病理学分会第十二届委员会病理学教学工作委员会委员，河北省医学会病理学分会委员，河北省医学会病理教学与教改学组副组长，唐山市医学会病理学分会副主任委员。发表论文 100 余篇（SCI 收录 20 余篇），主编著作 1 部，参编著作 3 部。主持与完成国家自然科学基金项目 1 项、省（部）及市（厅）级科研项目 8 项。获河北省教学成果一等奖 1 项，河北省科技进步二等奖 1 项、三等奖 2 项，中国煤炭工业科学技术三等奖 1 项。

编者简介

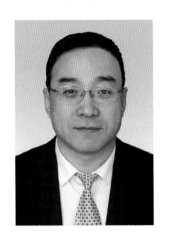

刘和亮

华北理工大学教授／主任医师，博士生导师。华北理工大学公共卫生学院院长，河北省器官纤维化重点实验室主任。河北省唐山市第十二届政协委员。中华预防医学会自由基预防医学专业委员会副主任委员，《中国煤炭工业医学杂志》主编，《南方医科大学学报》特邀编委。发表论文 100 余篇（SCI 收录 20 余篇）。在研国家自然科学基金项目 2 项，河北省重点研发项目和河北省自然科学基金项目各 1 项，完成省部级其他项目 5 项。获得国家教育部科技进步二等奖 1 项，省部级科技进步三等奖 1 项。

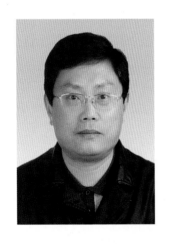

宋旭东

华北理工大学附属医院病理科主任，教授／主任医师，硕士生导师。中华医学会病理学分会尸检学组委员，北京肿瘤病理精准诊断研究会常委，北京肿瘤学会病理专业委员会第一届病理专业委员会常委，河北省预防学会第六届理事会理事，河北省医学会病理学分会第九届委员会常务委员，河北省医师协会病理科医师分会第三届委员会常委，河北省预防医学会分子病理与儿童疾病预防专业委员会第一届副主任委员，河北省中西医结合学会第一届病理专业委员会副主任委员。发表论文 60 余篇（SCI 收录 3 篇），主编图谱 1 部，参编著作 2 部。主持与完成市（厅）级科研项目 5 项，获唐山市科技进步一等奖、河北医学科技一等奖各 1 项，河北医学科技二等奖 3 项。

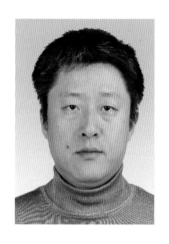

徐 洪

华北理工大学公共卫生学院副研究员,医学博士,硕士生导师。河北省"三三三人才工程"第三层次人选。河北省生理科学会第九届理事会理事、河北省抗癌协会肿瘤病因委员会委员。主持与完成国家自然科学基金项目 1 项、河北省自然科学基金项目 2 项、河北省研究生示范课程 1 项、河北省教育厅重点项目 1 项。获中国煤炭科技进步三等奖 1 项。发表 SCI 期刊论文 20 余篇。担任 *Molecular Therapy-Nucleic Acids*、*SCIENCE CHINA Life Sciences*、*Theranostics* 等学术期刊审稿人。

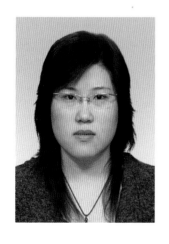

魏中秋

华北理工大学基础医学院讲师 / 医师,医学博士。主持与完成市科技局计划项目 1 项,河北省卫生计生委员会医学科学研究课题计划项目 1 项,参与国家自然科学基金面上项目 4 项。发表论文 60 余篇(SCI 收录 10 余篇),主编著作 2 部。获中国煤炭工业科学技术三等奖 1 项、河北省医学会二等奖 2 项。

余从事职业病临床工作已逾55年,虽倍感艰辛,不胜周折,却也不时收获成功和快乐。曾十分猖獗的传统职业危害(如中暑、铅、汞、锰、苯、砷窒息性或刺激性气体中毒等)基本上得到解决;不断出现的新化学因素危害(如有机溶剂,高分子化合物单体,铍、镉、铊等金属等)也逐次被攻克;不少临床研究(如新型金属络合剂二巯丁二酸、有机氟中毒、有机磷农药中毒、中毒性肾病、CO中毒迟发脑病、化学性急性呼吸窘迫综合征、亚急性二氯乙烷中毒性脑病、正己烷中毒性周围神经病、三氯乙烯药疹样皮炎、手臂震动病等)都有创新性发现,有力地推动了职业医学的发展。近一二十年,职业医学还积极响应社会需求,针对逐年增多的生活性中毒,以及各种化学事故、恐怖活动等,主动开展救治和研究,展示了职业医学强烈的社会责任心,得到了广大群众认可。但我国最主要的职业危害,约占我国职业病总数90%以上的尘肺病,确发病率持续不降,诊断手段滞后,治疗和康复仍在困境中摸索。

令人高兴的是,近十余年来,尘肺病临床困境已经引起广泛关注,一些现代化医学手段,如数字影像、计算机体层摄影、人工智能影像诊断、体液和支气管灌洗液检测(硅元素、细胞因子、酶等)、动态心肺功能联检、血气分析、基因诊断技术等,开始介入尘肺病诊断探索;尘肺肺纤维化治疗实验和临床研究也已启动,支气管或全肺灌洗、岩盐气溶胶吸入等手段均在改善症状和阻滞尘肺进展方面显示可喜前景;抗氧化措施、干细胞或核糖核酸干预、细胞因子治疗等实验研究已曙光初见;以抗炎、抗氧化、改善肺循环状况、活血化瘀为目标的中西医综合疗法在多中心的临床观察中也取得肯定疗效,不仅改善症状,且可显著消融各种肺纤维化病变,为尘肺病开辟了全新的临床前景。

今又有幸先睹杨方教授等主编的《煤工尘肺病理学图谱》,获益尤多!本书以占尘肺病80%以上的"煤工尘肺"为焦点,以47例具有完整临床和尸检资料的病例为研究材料,以病程为线索,汇集了近300幅并附有一些特殊染色的病理图像,清楚展示了各种病理改变的特点,分类更为精细,还附加许多大体形态学病变图像,更为全面、深刻地揭示了煤工尘肺的发病规律,对其他尘肺病也有重要启示。病理学是基础医学与临床医学间的桥梁,它通过疾病过程中机体功能和结构的变化,追索其与临床表现之间的关系,为阐明疾病本质,指导诊断、治疗和预防提供了可靠依据,无愧为"医生的医生"(doctor's doctor);本书丰富的内容无疑也将对尘肺病,尤其是煤工尘肺诊断治疗产生无可估量的积极作用。

"山不在高,有仙则名;水不在深,有龙则灵。"杨方教授等所在华北理工大学医学部的前身是华北煤炭医学院,50余年来一直致力于尘肺病的研究,蜚声国内外,该图谱乃是该校病理学团队长期攻关钻研的结晶,弥足珍贵。为编纂本书,该团队又在整理资料基础上,重新切片、染色、阅片、摄片,并配以中、英两种文字说明,展现了严谨负责的治学态度和认真求实的工作作风。本书篇幅虽然不大,但尽皆精粹,乃近年少见的学术佳作,值得向中外同道推荐;亦殷切期望作者勿忘初心,砥砺攀登,争取更大成绩,为祖国的卫生事业作出更大贡献!

北京大学第三医院职业病研究中心教授、博士生导师
赵金垣
2020 年 9 月

序 二

煤工尘肺（也称"煤矿尘肺"）是尘肺病的重要类型，为煤矿工人在生产过程中由于长期吸入悬浮在大气中的生产性粉尘所引起的尘肺病，是严重危害人民健康的职业病。煤工尘肺病发病机制复杂，病理形态多样，组织学类型上既可以形成煤矽肺、矽肺，也可以形成煤肺。患者即使脱离了粉尘作业的现场，病情仍持续进展。认识煤工尘肺的病理学变化特点是洞察其发生发展规律、优化现场针对性预防和指导临床合理治疗的基础。

华北理工大学病理学团队长期从事煤工尘肺的研究探索，研究工作历时50余年，前赴后继、与时俱进、持续深入，形成了特色鲜明的优势学术方向，研究成果在国内外同行中具有举足轻重的引领地位。本书是以杨方教授为首的老中青科学家基于华北理工大学病理学系47例煤工尘肺尸检标本材料的挖掘和创新，他们对尸检材料大体标本和组织切片进行了系统的整理和分析，增加了必要的免疫组化和特殊染色，从大量的图片资料中挑选出近300幅煤工尘肺典型病变图片，结合相关文字资料，形成了图文并茂的《煤工尘肺病理学图谱》。

本书的特点一是内容丰富全面，既有大体形态特点，又有组织学改变。从煤工尘肺的各种基本病变包括煤斑灶、煤矽结节、矽结节、块状纤维化等等，到肺实质和肺间质变化、淋巴结病变、胸膜病变、动脉管壁病变以及煤工尘肺伴发肺结核病、煤工尘肺伴发肺癌均有翔实的涵盖。图谱还附有部分典型的煤工尘肺案例，对不同期别的煤工尘肺及其合并症的病变进行了诠释；二是学术价值高，图片典型而精美，代表性好，直观揭示了煤工尘肺各种病理变化。图谱中还展示了大小不等、形状各异的煤尘灶图片，有助于增加读者兴趣，加深读者的印象；三是编撰方式系统性强，简明扼要的文字表述部分为读者了解煤工尘肺的发生发展、病理变化及转归奠定了知识基础，典型生动的图片作为核心要素，支撑了煤工尘肺病理变化的知识体系，文图并重，具有良好的知识性、可读性和实用性。

从获赐书稿到现在已一月有余,反复阅读,获益甚多。掩卷深思,感慨万千,作为一位从事病理事业多年的老兵,深深体会到了本书的珍贵。一是本书编撰人员对煤工尘肺防治事业学术坚持与奉献精神弥足珍贵,本书形成过程既有病理学界前辈李铁生教授和李洪珍教授等奠定的基础,更有杨方教授、刘和亮教授等近40年坚守煤工尘肺研究方向,孜孜以求、不断创新的努力。尤为可喜的是有孙影教授、宋旭东教授以及徐洪、魏中秋等学术新星的加入,为团队煤工尘肺研究进一步深入与提高奠定了坚实的人才基础。二是本书病理资料对煤工尘肺防治研究与临床实践的指导价值弥足珍贵,本书资料来源于国内较大宗的煤工尘肺尸检资料,涵盖煤工尘肺各期病例,并包括了煤工尘肺合并结核、肺癌和肺心病的资料,尽管由于年代久远个别肺腺癌图片不够十分理想,但瑕不掩瑜,在目前的环境下已经基本上不可能再获得此类资料,本书病理资料作为孤本资料对煤工尘肺防治的意义难以估价。

本书中英文双语撰写,既可作为工具书应用于本科、研究生的教学,也可作为参考资料指导职业病防治人员研究和临床实践。对于职业安全与管理人员的培训也是重要的教科书。

河北医科大学教授、博士生导师
张祥宏
2020 年 9 月

前　言

　　本书资料的大体与切片标本，来自华北理工大学(原华北煤炭医学院)病理学系尸检库存标本。20世纪70—80年代期间，在病理学系前辈李铁生教授和李洪珍教授的带领下，青年教师杨方、王献华、佟树文、张素华、张小萍、刘京跃、郑素琴、李琪佳等参加下，对47例来自内蒙古包头矿务局、内蒙古乌达矿务局、内蒙古渤海湾矿务局、山西霍县矿务局、山西阳泉矿务局、河北开滦矿务局、河北八宝山煤矿、湖南金竹山煤矿等矿区，较长时间从事煤矿井下工作的死亡矿工尸体或脏器进行解剖与诊断。年龄最小30岁，最大78岁，平均年龄为50.6岁，其中病理诊断尘肺Ⅰ期17例、Ⅱ期7例、Ⅲ期5例，无尘肺期(原称之为煤尘性反应期)18例。并留下了这批弥足珍贵的史料。这些史料的部分内容曾经以期刊论文的形式发表[1-11]，部分组织形态学内容也编辑出版了一部《煤矿尘肺病理组织学图谱》(黑白图片)[12]。但这批史料的大体标本形态学的内容以及组织形态学的一些内容尚未以彩色图片的形式进行编辑与发表。

　　我国是世界上最大的发展中国家，具有庞大的产业工人队伍，职业人群近8亿人，其中接触职业性有害因素的劳动者人数占劳动力的30%左右，约2亿多人[13]。我国目前正处于经济发展和社会转型期，一些传统的职业病，如尘肺病等尚未得到有效控制和解决。而且随着新技术、新材料的推广应用，也带来了一系列新的职业卫生问题，威胁着我国的公共卫生安全和经济安全[13-16]。我国有着丰富的煤炭资源，煤炭一直是我国主要的能源之一。目前，煤炭工业在我国国民经济中仍然占有十分重要的地位[17]。根据国家统计局第三次全国经济普查数据显示，截至2013年底中国煤炭行业从业人员总数达611.3万人，其中煤矿工人占比重最大。自2010年至2017年，尘肺病每年新发病例均超过2万例(其中90%以上为煤工尘肺和矽肺)，累计病例数已经达到83万余例[18,19]。而2019年5月国家卫生健康委员会发布的《2018年我国卫生健康事业发展统计公报》显示，2018年职业性尘肺新增病例为19 468例[20]。近年来，尘肺病发病呈现出持续高发、有所上升趋势，并出现患病年龄年轻化，发病时限缩短，并发症增多等一些新特点[22-29]。因此，尘肺病目前已经成为我国重大的职业卫生安全问题。然而，尘肺(包括煤工尘肺)病发病机制复杂，病理形态多样[1,3,5]。临床上即使患者脱离了粉尘作业的现场，但病情仍持续进展、病程迁延难愈，预后较差。因此对其形态学进行深入细致的观察，对于阐明煤工尘肺病理变化特点及其疾病发生、发展规律有着十分重要的意义。

　　尘肺病的研究是华北理工大学长期以来重点研究的课题，有着悠久的研究历史，并取得了丰富的研究成果，是华北理工大学的特色、优势学科建设的重要内容。本书是在整理、归纳了华北理工大学病理学系47例煤工尘肺尸检标本材料基础上,对其大体与切片标本进行了大体与显微镜的拍照,在数千张照片中挑选出近300幅典型病变图片,每张图片均标注了职业性接触煤尘的病史,并配以了中英文说明。此书是在继承《煤矿尘肺组织学图谱》总体风格的基础上,做了较多的补充。彩色图片的效果也进一步补遗了黑白照片的一些瑕疵,一些特殊染色(Masson、免疫组化、天狼星红等染色)[30-36],使病变特点体现得更加清楚与明晰。同时也参考了《尘肺病理诊断图谱》一书的一些内容[37],附有部分典型的煤工尘肺案例,对不同期别的煤工尘肺及其合并症的病变进行了诠释。

对这些史料的重新挖掘、整理、编辑与发表,使史料再次彰显了科研与教学的双重效益,历久弥新、展示出不同寻常的科学与实用价值。

此书,不仅适用于本科、研究生的教学,同时对于从事职业病研究领域的研究生及其科研工作者也是很好的学习、参考资料。对于职业安全与管理人员的培训无疑也是重要的教科书。此书图谱采用中英文双语标注,便于留学生教学与国际合作与交流。

在编写过程中,孙影教授对史料的保存、挖掘、整理与英文的编辑做了卓有成效的工作。刘和亮教授在书籍的策划与编写过程中给予了很好的建议。宋旭东教授在肺部疾病诊断,尤其是煤工尘肺合并结核病、肿瘤病变的病理形态诊断方面给予了认真细致的观察与分析。徐洪副研究员在切片补充过程中,对一些特殊染色方法的改良与实施做出了重要贡献。魏中秋博士在对大体标本与切片标本的修复、整理、挑选与拍照过程付出了较多的心血与汗水。杨方教授负责本书的整体策划,并对大体标本的挑选、切片标本的拍照及其编辑做了大量具体细致的工作。此外,每位编者对各自负责的章节进行了认真编写,使这本具有"乌金"色彩的图谱能够奉献给广大的读者。

此书在编写过程中不免存在一些缺陷和诸多不足之处,敬请同行与读者给予批评指正。

编　者
2020 年 9 月

Preface

All involved samples are from the precious collection of pathology department of North China University of Science and Technology (formerly known as North China Coal Medical College). Back to 1970s, Chinese famous pathologists Tie-Sheng Li and Hong-Zhen Li, leading their research team (including Fang Yang, Xian-Hua Wang, Shu-Wen Tong, Su-Hua Zhang, Xiao-Ping Zhang, Jing-Yue Liu, Su-Qin Zheng, Qi-Jia Li) spend nearly 20 years in studying death causes and pathogenesis of coal workers' pneumoconiosis, based on 47 cases who had been in coal mine industries for a long time (The industries include Baotou mining bureau of Inner Mongolia autonomous region, Wuda mining bureau of Inner Mongolia autonomous region, Bohaiwan mining bureau of Inner Mongolia autonomous region, Huoxian mining bureau of Shanxi province, Yangquan mining bureau of Shanxi province, Kaiping mining bureau of Hebei province, Jinzhushan mining bureau of Hunan province, Babaoshan mining bureau of Hebei province.). Age of 47 cases ranges from 30 years old to 78 years old, with an average age of 50.6 years old. All cases are definitely diagnosed with coal workers' pneumoconiosis, including stage I (17 cases), stage II (7 cases), stage III (5 cases), no pneumoconiosis stage (formerly known as coal dust reaction stage, 18 cases). Although the documents have published some of precious research outcomes[1-11], and the book (*Histological Atlas of Coal Mine Pneumoconiosis*) has facilitated partial histological photographs (in black and white) presentation[12], it keeps a pity that much of the morphological information has undiscovered.

China is the largest developing country, with a population accounting for 800 millions of industrial workers, 30% of whom (more than 200 million workers) are exposed to occupational harmful factors[13]. Nowadays, China has migrated into the transition period for the industrial aspect. Some of traditional occupational diseases, such as pneumoconiosis, are still in the situation of hard controlling and therapy, and the new occupational health problems arise due to the application of new technologies and new materials, being a big problem about public health safety and economic security[13-16]. China is rich in coal resource which plays an important supportive role in energies consumption and national economy[17]. The third national economic census in China, illustrates 6.113 million of employees working in coal mine industry by the end of 2013, most of which are coal miners. From 2010, it is eight consecutive years that the new cases are higher than 20,000 each year, more than 90% of which is coal workers' pneumoconiosis and silicosis. Therefore, there are more than 830,000 cases of coal workers' pneumoconiosis in total[18,19]. According to a statistics communique recently released by the National Health Commission, 19,468 new cases arise only in 2018[20]. Moreover, pneumoconiosis is appended with the new characteristics, such as a high incidence of pneumoconiosis, younger age, shortened latency and increased complications, growing a big problem about occupational health and safety [22-29]. However, the pathogenesis of pneumoconiosis (including coal worker's pneumoconiosis) is complex, varying in pathological changes [1,3,5]. In clinic, pneumoconiosis is continuously progressive, therapy keeping no effective and prognosis being poor even in the patients who have no exposure to silica for a long time. Therefore, details of pathological changes have a great contribution on discovering pathogenesis and development law of coal worker's pneumoconiosis.

North China University of Science and Technology has been studying pneumoconiosis for several decades, receiving substantial achievements. Based on 47 cases of autopsy specimens, this book carefully collects close to 300 photographs from several thousands of morphological images, showing the typical gross appearances and histological changes, denoting with instructions in English Chinese and medical history. It is not only a renew of *Histological Atlas of Coal Mine Pneumoconiosis*, but also a great improvement in presentation ways, such as photographs in color, application of special staining (Masson, Immunohistochemistry, Sirius red) [30-36]. In the part of attachment, this book employs seven clinical cases to further elucidate the pathological changes and complications of coal worker's pneumoconiosis [37].

The presentation of these precious historical outcomes facilitates might manifest its great practical value in both scientific research and medical education. This book is suitable for not only undergraduate and graduate students, but also the scientists who study in the field of occupational diseases. It provides the benefits in occupational safety and management. The version in both English and Chinese is convenient for international students learning and international communication.

The book is the joint efforts of all of colleagues. Professor Ying Sun has a contribution on preservation of these precious historical outcomes and English annotation. Professor He-Liang Liu provides many excellent suggestions. Professor Xu-Dong Song performs the careful observation and analysis in coal worker's pneumoconiosis with tuberculosis and lung cancer. Hong Xu, associate research fellow, makes a great contribution on improvement of special staining. Dr. Zhong-Qiu Wei strives in repairing these precious specimens, taking and picking up classic photographs. Professor Yang fang is in charge of managing all workload, epically in the overall plan, and photographs collection.

There are still some defects in this book. We would appreciate your comments and suggestions.

Authors

September,2020

图　谱　导　读

第一部分　肺脏的基本结构与形态学特点

1　肺脏的解剖学 ··· 2
2　肺脏的组织形态学 ·· 3
　2.1　肺实质：导气部和呼吸部 ·· 3
　2.2　肺间质：肺的血管、淋巴管和神经组织 ······························· 6

第二部分　煤工尘肺形态学特点

1　煤工尘肺大体形态学特点 ··· 8
　1.1　煤斑灶：包括胸膜煤斑灶和肺内煤斑灶 ······························· 8
　　1.1.1　胸膜煤斑灶 ··· 8
　　1.1.2　肺内煤斑灶 ··· 9
　1.2　结节病变 ·· 9
　　1.2.1　煤（矽）结节（即煤矽结节） ·································· 9
　　1.2.2　矽（煤）结节（即矽结节） ·································· 9
　1.3　块状纤维化 ·· 9
　　1.3.1　进行性块状纤维化 ··· 9
　　1.3.2　结节融合型块状纤维化 ·· 9
　　1.3.3　混合型块状纤维化 ··· 9
　1.4　弥漫性间质纤维化 ··· 9
　1.5　肺气肿病变 ·· 9
　1.6　淋巴结的病变（多见肺门淋巴结的累及） ·························· 10
　1.7　胸膜病变 ·· 10
　1.8　煤工尘肺伴发肺结核病 ·· 10
　　1.8.1　煤斑灶伴粟粒性播散性肺结核 ································· 10

　　　1.8.2　块状纤维化伴粟粒性播散性肺结核 ………………………………………10
　　　1.8.3　煤工尘肺伴肺门淋巴结结核病变 …………………………………………10
　1.9　煤工尘肺伴发肺癌 ……………………………………………………………………10
　　　1.9.1　煤工尘肺伴结节型肺癌 …………………………………………………10
　　　1.9.2　煤工尘肺伴弥漫型肺癌 …………………………………………………10
　1.10　煤工尘肺伴发肺源性心脏病 ………………………………………………………10
2　煤工尘肺组织形态学特点 ………………………………………………………………10
　2.1　煤矽肺 ………………………………………………………………………………10
　　　2.1.1　煤斑(coal dust dots,区别于大体的煤斑灶 coal dust maculae) ………10
　　　2.1.2　煤尘灶 ………………………………………………………………………11
　　　2.1.3　结节病变 ……………………………………………………………………11
　　　2.1.4　煤尘性块状纤维化 …………………………………………………………12
　　　2.1.5　煤尘性间质纤维化 …………………………………………………………12
　2.2　矽煤肺(矽肺) ………………………………………………………………………12
　　　2.2.1　巨噬细胞性肺泡炎 …………………………………………………………12
　　　2.2.2　矽(煤)结节(又称矽结节) ………………………………………………12
　　　2.2.3　矽肺块状纤维化 ……………………………………………………………12
　　　2.2.4　尘性间质纤维化 ……………………………………………………………13
　2.3　煤肺 …………………………………………………………………………………13
　2.4　伴发性病变 …………………………………………………………………………13
　　　2.4.1　合并肺结核病 ………………………………………………………………13
　　　2.4.2　合并肺肿瘤 …………………………………………………………………14
　2.5　其他病变 ……………………………………………………………………………14
　　　2.5.1　淋巴结的病变 ………………………………………………………………14
　　　2.5.2　支气管的累及与病变 ………………………………………………………14
　　　2.5.3　胸膜的累及与病变 …………………………………………………………15
　　　2.5.4　煤尘性肺气肿 ………………………………………………………………15
　　　2.5.5　小血管的累及与病变 ………………………………………………………15
　　　2.5.6　脂肪组织的累及 ……………………………………………………………15
　　　2.5.7　淋巴管的累及 ………………………………………………………………15
　　　2.5.8　神经纤维的累及 ……………………………………………………………15
　　　2.5.9　肺内继发各种感染性病变 …………………………………………………15
　　　2.5.10　棒状小体(含铁小体) ……………………………………………………15
　　　2.5.11　肌成纤维细胞分化 …………………………………………………………15
　　　2.5.12　肺源性心脏病 ……………………………………………………………16
参考文献 ……………………………………………………………………………………16

Contents

Atlas Guide

Part I   Anatomy and Histology of Lung

1 Anatomy of the lung ··· 20
2 Histology of the lung ··· 21
   2.1 Parenchyma: It includes conduction portion and respiratory portion ··············· 21
   2.2 Mesenchyma: It contains blood vessels, lymphatic vessels and nerves ············· 25

Part II   Pathology of Coal Workers' Pneumoconiosis

1 Gross appearance of coal workers' pneumoconiosis ································· 27
   1.1 Coal dust maculae ··· 27
      1.1.1 Pleural coal dust maculae ··· 28
      1.1.2 Pulmonary coal dust maculae ·· 28
   1.2 Coal dust nodules ··· 28
      1.2.1 Coal (silicotic) nodules (coal silicotic nodules) ······························· 28
      1.2.2 Silicotic (coal) nodules (silicotic nodules) ······································ 28
   1.3 Massive fibrosis ··· 28
      1.3.1 Progressive massive fibrosis ··· 28
      1.3.2 Nodular confluent massive fibrosis ·· 28
      1.3.3 Combination of progressive massive fibrosis and nodular confluent massive
           fibrosis ··· 29
   1.4 Diffuse interstitial fibrosis ·· 29
   1.5 Emphysema ·· 29
   1.6 Lesions in the lymph nodes (usually in hilar lymph nodes) ·························· 29
   1.7 Lesions in pleura ·· 29
   1.8 Coal works' pneumoconiosis with tuberculosis ·· 29

    1.8.1   Coal dust maculae with disseminated miliary tuberculosis ·················· 29

    1.8.2   Massive fibrosis with disseminated miliary tuberculosis ····················· 29

    1.8.3   Coal works' pneumoconiosis with tuberculosis in hilar lymph nodes ············ 30

1.9   Coal works' pneumoconiosis with lung cancer ··································· 30

    1.9.1   Coal works' pneumoconiosis with lung cancer (Peripheral type) ················ 30

    1.9.2   Coal works' pneumoconiosis with lung cancer (Diffuse type) ·················· 30

1.10   Coal works' pneumoconiosis with cor pulmonale ···························· 30

2 Histological changes of coal workers' pneumoconiosis ······························ 30

2.1 Anthracosilicosis ·· 30

    2.1.1   Coal dust dots ·· 30

    2.1.2   Coal dust foci ·· 30

    2.1.3   Nodular lesion ·· 31

    2.1.4   Massive fibrosis ··· 32

    2.1.5   Coal interstitial fibrosis ······································ 32

2.2 Silicosis ·· 32

    2.2.1   Macrophage alveolitis ·· 32

    2.2.2   Silicotic (coal) nodules (silicotic nodules) ·························· 32

    2.2.3   Massive fibrosis ··· 33

    2.2.4   Dust interstitial fibrosis ······································· 33

2.3 Anthracosis ··· 33

2.4 Complicated lesions ·· 34

    2.4.1   Pulmonary tuberculosis ······································· 34

    2.4.2   Lung tumor ··· 34

2.5 Others ··· 35

    2.5.1   Lesions of lymph nodes ······································· 35

    2.5.2   Lesions of bronchi ··· 35

    2.5.3   Lesions of pleura ··· 36

    2.5.4   Emphysema in response to coal dust ······························ 36

    2.5.5   Lesions of small blood vessels ··································· 36

    2.5.6   Lesions of adipose tissue ······································ 36

    2.5.7   Lesions of lymphatic vessels ···································· 36

    2.5.8   Lesions of nerves ··· 36

    2.5.9   Pulmonary infection ··· 36

    2.5.10   "Rod-shaped" body ·· 37

    2.5.11   Myofibroblast differentiation ··································· 37

    2.5.12   Cor pulmonale ·· 37

References ·· 37

图谱部分 Atlas

第一部分　煤工尘肺大体形态学特点

Part I　Gross Appearance of Coal Workers' Pneumoconiosis

图 1　胸膜煤斑灶··43

Fig.1　Pleural coal dust maculae ···43

图 2 至图 4　肺内煤斑灶··43

Fig.2 to Fig.4　Pulmonary coal dust maculae··43

图 5　肺内煤斑灶伴大泡型肺气肿形成···45

Fig.5　Pulmonary coal dust maculae accompanied by bullous emphysema ·····45

图 6　肺内煤斑灶伴囊泡型肺气肿形成···45

Fig.6　Pulmonary coal dust maculae with cystic emphysema ·····················45

图 7 和图 8　肺内煤斑灶（全肺大切片标本）···46

Fig.7 and Fig.8　Pulmonary coal dust maculae（the large slice）···················46

图 9 和图 10　肺内煤斑灶（肺叶大切片标本）··47

Fig.9 and Fig.10　Pulmonary coal dust maculae（the large slice）··················47

图 11 和图 12　肺内煤斑灶、煤尘纤维灶（煤结节）形成·······························48

Fig.11 and Fig.12　Pulmonary coal dust maculae and fibrotic lesions（coal dust nodule）·········48

图 13 和图 14　肺内煤斑灶、煤矽结节··49

Fig.13 and Fig.14　Pulmonary coal dust maculae and coal silicotic nodules ·····49

图 15 和图 16　肺内煤斑灶、煤矽结节··50

Fig.15 and Fig.16　Pulmonary coal dust maculae and coal silicotic nodules ·····50

图 17 和图 18　肺内煤斑灶··51

Fig.17 and Fig.18　Pulmonary coal dust maculae ······································51

图 19 和图 20　进行性块状纤维化··52

Fig.19 and Fig.20　Progressive massive fibrosis·······································52

图 21 和图 22　进行性块状纤维化（肺大切片标本）······································53

Fig.21 and Fig.22　Progressive massive fibrosis（the large slice）··················53

图 23 和图 24　结节融合型块状纤维化··54

Fig.23 and Fig.24　Nodular confluent massive fibrosis ·······························54

图 25 和图 26　结节融合型块状纤维化（同图 23 肺大切片标本）······················55

Fig.25 and Fig.26　Nodular confluent massive fibrosis（this large slice shares the sample with Fig.23）···55

图 27 和图 28　混合型块状纤维化···56

Fig.27 and Fig.28　Mixed massive fibrosis ···56

图 29 至图 38　煤工尘肺伴结核病···57

Fig.29 to Fig.38　Coal works' pneumoconiosis with tuberculosis ················57

图 39　煤工尘肺伴肺癌（周围型）···62

Fig.39　Coal works' pneumoconiosis with lung cancer（Peripheral type）········62

图 40　煤工尘肺伴肺癌（弥漫型）···62

Fig.40　Coal works' pneumoconiosis with lung cancer（Diffuse type）·········62

图 41 和图 42　煤工尘肺伴胸膜粘连与增厚··63

Fig.41 and Fig.42　Coal works' pneumoconiosis with pleural adhesion and thickening ··········63

图 43 和图 44　煤工尘肺合并肺源性心脏病··64

Fig.43 and Fig.44　Coal works' pneumoconiosis with cor pulmonale ············64

第二部分　煤工尘肺组织形态学特点

Part II　Histological Appearance of Coal Workers' Pneumoconiosis

图 45 至图 48　胸膜煤斑··66

Fig.45 to Fig.48　Coal dust dots of pleura ···66

图 49 至图 52　肺内煤斑··68

Fig.49 to Fig.52　Coal dust dots of lung ···68

图 53 和图 54　煤尘细胞灶···70

Fig.53 and Fig.54　Cellular coal dust foci ···70

图 55 至图 58　煤尘纤维灶···71

Fig.55 to Fig.58　Fibrous coal dust foci ··71

图 59 至图 74　大小不等、形状各异的煤尘灶···73

Fig.59 to Fig.74　Coal dust lesions varying in size and shape ·····················73

图 75 至图 78　巨噬细胞性肺泡炎···77

Fig.75 to Fig.78　Macrophage alveolitis ··77

图 79 至图 82　煤尘细胞性结节···79

Fig.79 to Fig.82　Cellular coal dust nodules ···79

图 83 至图 86　细胞纤维性结节···81

Fig.83 to Fig.86　Cellular fibrous nodules ···81

图 87 至图 94　煤矽结节··83

Fig.87 to Fig.94　Coal silicotic nodules ··83

图 95　不典型煤矽结节··88

Fig.95　Atypical coal silicotic nodule ···88

图 96 至图 103　融合型煤矽结节···89

Fig.96 to Fig.103　Confluent coal silicotic nodules ·································· 89

图 104　矽结节·· 93

Fig.104　Silicotic nodule·· 93

图 105　融合型矽结节··· 93

Fig.105　Confluent silicotic nodules ·· 93

图 106 至图 109　矽结节·· 94

Fig.106 to Fig.109　Silicotic nodule ·· 94

图 110 至图 113　进行性块状纤维化·· 96

Fig.110 to Fig.113　Progressive massive fibrosis ·· 96

图 114 和图 115　融合型块状纤维化·· 98

Fig.114 and Fig.115　Confluent massive fibrous lesion ·································· 98

图 116 和图 117　弥漫性尘性间质纤维化·· 99

Fig.116 and Fig.117　Diffuse coal interstitial fibrosis···································· 99

图 118 和图 119　间质纤维化伴平滑肌细胞局灶性增生································· 100

Fig.118 and Fig.119　Interstitial fibrosis with local proliferated smooth muscle cells ······ 100

图 120 和图 121　煤工尘肺伴结核病变·· 101

Fig.120 and Fig.121　Coal workers' pneumoconiosis with tuberculosis ············· 101

图 122　肺内早期煤矽结核结节·· 102

Fig.122　Early stage of coal silicotic tuberculous nodule ······························ 102

图 123　肺内典型的煤矽结核结节··· 102

Fig.123　Classic coal silicotic tuberculous nodule ······································ 102

图 124　肺内煤矽结核结节·· 103

Fig.124　Coal silicotic tuberculous nodules ··· 103

图 125 至图 127　肺内融合型煤矽结核结节··· 103

Fig.125 to Fig.127　Confluent coal silicotic tuberculous nodules····················· 103

图 128 和图 129　煤工尘肺矽结核结节·· 105

Fig.128 and Fig.129　Silicotic tuberculous nodules of coal works' pneumoconiosis·········· 105

图 130　结节融合型块状纤维化··· 106

Fig.130　Nodular confluent massive fibrosis ··· 106

图 131 至图 134　煤工尘肺伴播散性粟粒性肺结核·· 106

Fig.131 to Fig.134　Disseminated miliary tuberculosis of coal workers' pneumoconiosis······ 106

图 135　尘性结核性结节·· 108

Fig.135　Coal dust tuberculous nodules ·· 108

图 136 和图 137　尘性结核性肉芽肿(结节)··· 109

Fig.136 and Fig.137　Coal dust tuberculous granuloma（nodule）····················· 109

图 138 和图 139　尘性结核性支气管炎·· 110

Fig.138 and Fig.139　Coal dust tuberculous bronchiolitis ····························· 110

图 140　煤工尘肺伴结核性胸膜炎··· 111

Fig.140　Tuberculous pleuritis of coal workers' pneumoconiosis ····················· 111

图 141 煤工尘肺结核性空洞···111

Fig. 141 Tuberculous cavity of coal workers' pneumoconiosis ···············111

图 142 和图 143 煤工尘肺伴发肺腺癌··112

Fig.142 and Fig.143 Coal workers' pneumoconiosis with pulmonary adenocarcinoma········112

图 144 和图 145 煤工尘肺伴淋巴结转移腺癌·································113

Fig.144 and Fig.145 Coal workers' pneumoconiosis with lymph node adenocarcinoma
metastasis ···113

图 146 和图 147 煤工尘肺伴发肺腺癌··114

Fig.146 and Fig.147 Coal workers' pneumoconiosis with pulmonary adenocarcinoma········114

图 148 至图 151 煤工尘肺伴发腺鳞癌··115

Fig.148 to Fig.151 Coal workers' pneumoconiosis with pulmonary adenosquamous
carcinoma ···115

图 152 和图 153 煤工尘肺伴发恶性间皮瘤······································117

Fig.152 and Fig.153 Coal workers' pneumoconiosis with malignant mesothelioma········117

图 154 煤工尘肺伴发恶性间皮瘤淋巴结转移·······························118

Fig.154 Coal workers' pneumoconiosis with lymph node malignant mesothelioma
metastasis ···118

图 155 血管内瘤栓形成··118

Fig.155 Carcinoma cells emboli in small blood vessels ·····················118

图 156 至图 159 淋巴结煤尘沉积··119

Fig.156 to Fig.159 Lymph nodes with coal dust deposition ·················119

图 160 至图 163 淋巴结内煤矽结节··121

Fig.160 to Fig.163 Coal silicotic nodules in lymph nodes ··················121

图 164 淋巴结病变··123

Fig.164 Silicotic lesions in lymph nodes ·····································123

图 165 至图 167 淋巴结内矽结节··123

Fig.165 to Fig.167 Silicotic nodules in lymph node ························123

图 168 至图 171 淋巴结内融合型矽结节··125

Fig.168 to Fig.171 Confluent silicotic nodules in lymph node ···········125

图 172 和图 173 淋巴结内煤矽结核结节··127

Fig.172 and Fig.173 Coal silicotic tuberculous nodules in lymph nodes ···127

图 174 和图 175 淋巴结内矽结核结节··128

Fig.174 and Fig.175 Silicotic tuberculous nodules in lymph nodes ·······128

图 176 至图 180 煤尘侵及支气管··129

Fig.176 to Fig.180 Coal dust deposition in bronchi·······················129

图 181 至图 183 尘性慢性细支气管炎··131

Fig.181 to Fig.183 Coal chronic bronchiolitis ····························131

图 184 至图 189 胸膜病变··133

Fig. 814 to Fig.189 Pleural lesions ···133

图 190　煤尘沉积在肺内小支气管 ……………………………………………………136

Fig.190　Coal dust deposition in small bronchia ………………………………………136

图 191　煤尘沉积在肺内细支气管及终末细支气管 ……………………………………136

Fig.191　Coal dust deposition in small bronchia and terminal bronchia ………………136

图 192 和图 193　煤尘沉积在呼吸性细支气管及其分支 …………………………………137

Fig.192 and Fig.193　Coal dust deposition in respiratory bronchia and its branaches …………137

图 194　尘性小叶中心型肺气肿 ……………………………………………………………138

Fig.194　Coal dust-induced centriacinar emphysema ……………………………………138

图 195　全小叶破坏型肺气肿 ………………………………………………………………138

Fig.195　Destructive panacinar emphysema ………………………………………………138

图 196 和图 197　累及肺动脉 ………………………………………………………………139

Fig.196 and Fig.197　Lesions in pulmonary artery ………………………………………139

图 198　肺内小动脉病变 ……………………………………………………………………140

Fig.198　Lesions in pulmonary small arteries ……………………………………………140

图 199　肺内小血管病变 ……………………………………………………………………140

Fig.199　Lesions in pulmonary small vessels ……………………………………………140

图 200 和图 201　小动脉病变 ………………………………………………………………141

Fig.200 and Fig.201　Lesions in small arteries …………………………………………141

图 202　煤尘累及淋巴结及其脂肪组织 ……………………………………………………142

Fig.202　Coal dust deposits involve lymph nodes and adipose tissue …………………142

图 203　煤尘累及支气管及其周围脂肪组织 ………………………………………………142

Fig.203　Involvement of bronchi and adjacent fat tissue by coal dusts …………………142

图 204 和图 205　淋巴管病变 ………………………………………………………………143

Fig.204 and Fig.205　Lesions in the lymphatic vessels …………………………………143

图 206 和图 207　胸膜下神经纤维受累 ……………………………………………………144

Fig.206 and Fig.207　Coal dusts involve subpleural nerve fibers ………………………144

图 208　煤工尘肺伴浆液出血性炎 …………………………………………………………145

Fig.208　Coal workers' pneumoconiosis with serous hemorrhagic inflammation ………145

图 209　煤工尘肺伴肺水肿 …………………………………………………………………145

Fig.209　Coal workers' pneumoconiosis with pulmonary edema ………………………145

图 210 和图 211　煤工尘肺伴肺淤血、肺水肿 ……………………………………………146

Fig.210 and Fig.211　Coal workers' pneumoconiosis with pulmonary congestion and
　　　　　　　edema ………………………………………………………………………146

图 212　煤工尘肺伴化脓性炎 ………………………………………………………………147

Fig.212　Coal workers pneumoconiosis with purulent inflammation ……………………147

图 213　煤工尘肺伴脓肿 ……………………………………………………………………147

Fig.213　Coal workers' pneumoconiosis with abscess ……………………………………147

图 214　煤工尘肺伴浆液、纤维素性炎 ……………………………………………………148

Fig.214　Coal workers' pneumoconiosis with serous fibrinous inflammation ……………148

图 215　煤工尘肺伴浆液、化脓性炎 ··· 148

Fig.215　Coal workers' pneumoconiosis with serous purulent inflammation ············· 148

图 216 和图 217　煤工尘肺"棒状小体"形成 ··· 149

Fig.216 and Fig.217　"Rod-shaped" bodies of coal workers' pneumoconiosis ············ 149

图 218 至图 223　肌成纤维细胞分化 ··· 150

Fig.218 to Fig.223　Myofibroblasts differentiation ··· 150

图 224　正常心肌组织（右心室） ·· 154

Fig.224　Normal heart tissue（from right ventricle） ·· 154

图 225　肺源性心脏病心肌组织（右心室） ·· 154

Fig.225　Right ventricle with cor pulmonale ··· 154

第三部分　煤工尘肺案例

Part III　Cases of Coal Workers' Pneumoconiosis

案例一　煤矽肺Ⅰ期（结节＋尘斑 - 气肿） ·· 156

Case 1　Anthracosilicosis（stage Ⅰ, Nodules and maculae surrounded by emphysema）········· 157

案例二　煤肺Ⅰ期（煤尘斑灶＋细胞性结节） ·· 161

Case 2　Anthracosis（stage Ⅰ, Coal dust maculae and cellular nodules）················· 162

案例三　煤矽肺Ⅱ期（尘斑 - 气肿型） ·· 166

Case 3　Anthracosilicosis（stage Ⅱ, Coal dust maculae and emphysema）················· 167

案例四　煤矽肺Ⅲ期（大块纤维化） ··· 170

Case 4　Anthracosilicosis（stage Ⅲ, Massive fibrosis）···································· 171

案例五　煤矽肺Ⅲ期合并肺结核病 ·· 176

Case 5　Anthracosilicosis（stage Ⅲ）with pulmonary tuberculosis ······················ 177

案例六　煤矽肺Ⅲ期合并肺癌 ·· 182

Case 6　Anthracosilicosis（stage Ⅲ）with lung cancer ···································· 183

案例七　煤肺Ⅰ期（煤斑 - 气肿）合并肺源性心脏 ··· 189

Case 7　Anthracosis（stage Ⅰ, Coal dust maculae and emphysema）with cor pulmonale ········· 191

后记 ··· 198

Acknowledgement ·· 199

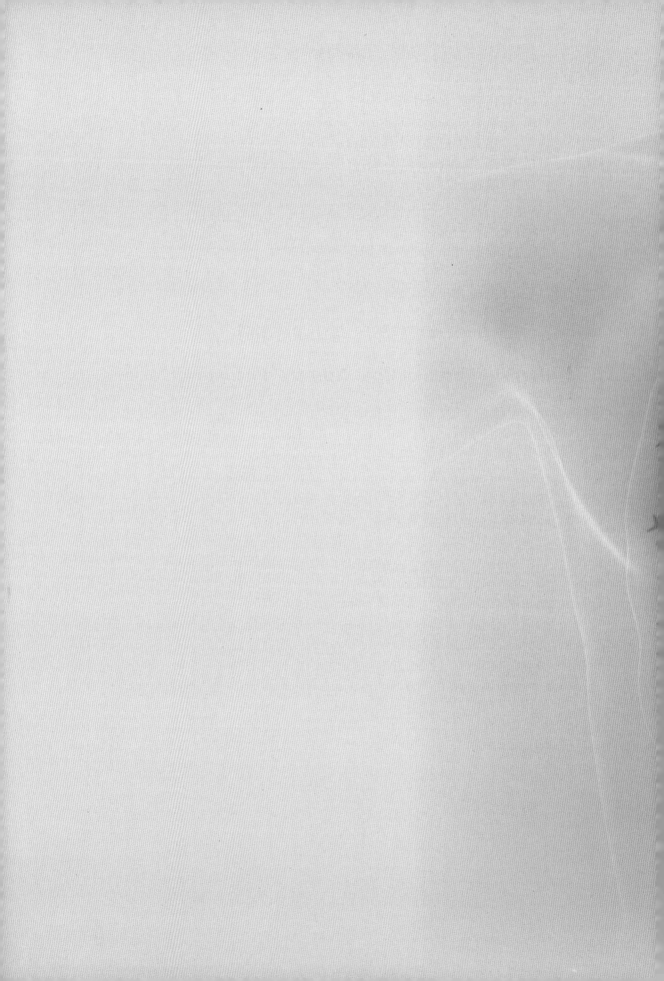

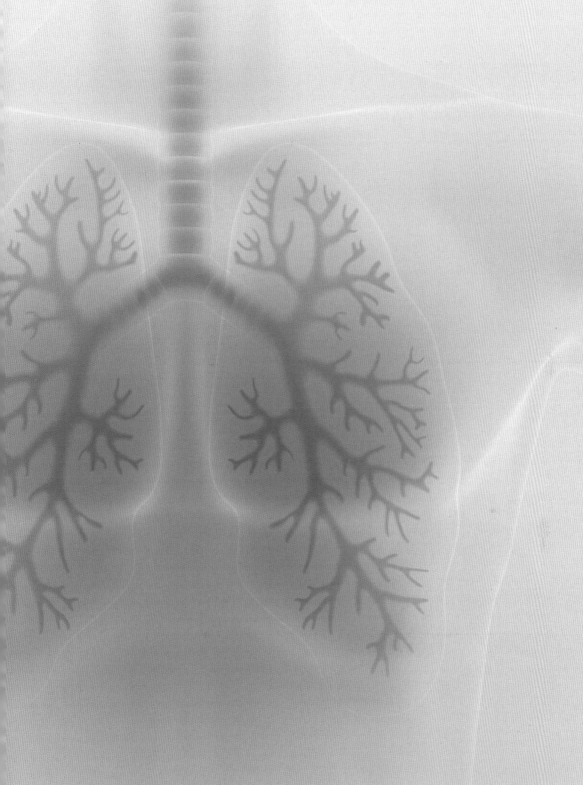

图谱导读

肺脏的基本结构与形态学特点[38,39]

1 肺脏的解剖学

　　肺脏位于胸腔,左、右肺分居纵隔两侧、膈肌之上。一般情况下,左肺由叶间裂(斜裂)分为上下两叶。右肺被斜裂和水平裂分为上中下三叶(图1)。

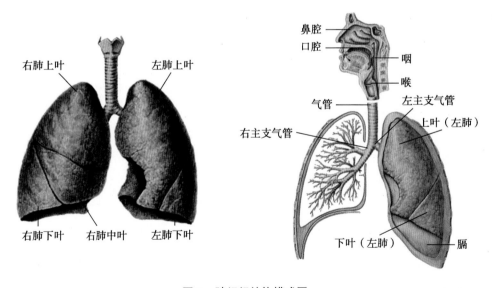

右肺上叶　左肺上叶

右肺下叶　右肺中叶　左肺下叶

鼻腔
口腔
咽
喉
气管　左主支气管
右主支气管　上叶(左肺)
下叶(左肺)　膈

图1　肺组织结构模式图

　　气管与支气管是连接肺之间的管道,由软骨、肌肉、黏膜和结缔组织构成。左、右支气管在肺门处分出肺叶支气管。肺叶支气管入肺后再分为肺段支气管,此后反复分支,呈树枝状,称之为支气管树。

支气管分支可达 25 级左右,直至连于肺泡。肺段支气管是支气管的第三级分支,每一个肺段均呈圆锥形,尖指向肺门。相邻肺段间有薄层结缔组织分隔。被视为肺的独立结构与功能单位。

肺段包含若干个肺小叶,所以肺小叶是我们能够肉眼看到的最小肺单位。肺小叶大小不等,一般在 1cm 左右的范围,为多面形锥体,锥体尖部处是细支气管与血管、淋巴管进入小叶的门户。小叶间有明显的结缔组织间隔,因此小叶间的周界是比较清楚的。

2　肺脏的组织形态学

肺组织分为实质与间质两部分。实质部分即肺内各级支气管和肺泡,间质部分为肺内的结缔组织、血管、淋巴管和神经等。

2.1　肺实质:导气部和呼吸部

2.1.1　导气部:为气体出入的部分。主支气管由肺门进入肺后,反复多次分支。由叶、段支气管分支之后,统称小支气管。小支气管分支至管径 1mm 以下时,则称为细支气管。细支气管再分支,管径达 0.5mm 以下时,称终末细支气管。即支气管至终末细支气管部分为肺的导气部。

肺内各级支气管随着管道分支,管径越来越细,管壁越来越薄,管壁的组织结构也随之发生相应的变化。

(1) 肺内支气管和小支气管(图 2)

1) 黏膜层:分为上皮与固有层。

上皮:假复层纤毛柱状上皮。其间夹杂杯状细胞。

固有层:位于上皮下的薄层致密结缔组织,包括少量胶原和较多弹力纤维。其外为平滑肌构成的黏膜肌层。

2) 黏膜下层:疏松结缔组织。其内含有少量腺体,为分泌黏液和浆液的混合腺体。

3) 外膜:结缔组织、透明软骨片。还有血管、淋巴管、神经等。

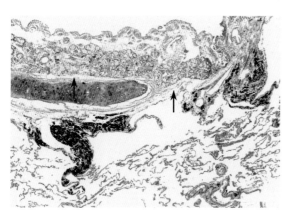
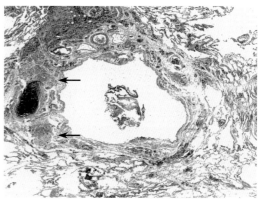

图 2　肺内小支气管结构(煤工尘肺):黏液腺体增生(箭头所指)

（2）细支气管（图3）

1）黏膜层

上皮：假复层或单层纤毛柱状上皮，其间夹杂少量杯状细胞。

固有层：薄，黏膜肌层的平滑肌相对增多，但尚未环绕成层。

2）黏膜下层：薄，有少量腺体或无腺体。

3）外膜：透明软骨片变小、减少或消失。含有血管、淋巴管、神经等。

（3）终末细支气管（图3）

1）黏膜层：

上皮：单层纤毛柱状上皮，无杯状细胞。

固有层：薄，平滑肌相对增多，环绕成层。

2）黏膜下层：薄，腺体消失。

3）外膜：无透明软骨片。含少量血管、淋巴管、神经等。

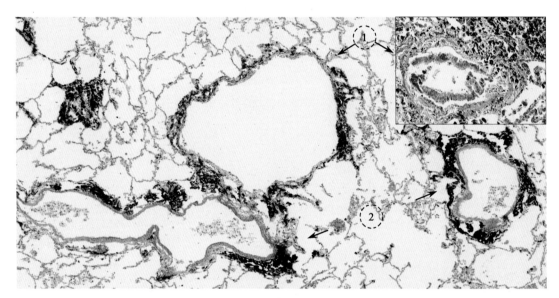

图3　细支气管与终末细支气管（煤工尘肺）：煤尘沉积在细支气管与终末细支气管

1- 细支气管：黏膜固有层平滑肌未形成层状环绕；2- 终末细支气管：固有层平滑肌层状环绕。

2.2.2　呼吸部：由呼吸性细支气管、肺泡管、肺泡囊和肺泡组成。

（1）呼吸性细支气管：是终末细支气管的分支。每个终末细支气管可分出两个或以上的呼吸性细支气管（图4）。

1）上皮：与终末细支气管相连接处为单层柱状纤毛上皮，向后逐渐移行为单层柱状、单层立方状上皮。在接近肺泡部分则逐渐转变为单层扁平上皮。

2）固有膜：很薄，含少量结缔组织和平滑肌。因为管道与肺泡相连，具有呼吸功能，故称呼吸性细支气管。

（2）肺泡管：为呼吸性细支气管连续3级分支后移行于肺泡管。其管壁有密集的肺泡开口。此处上皮为立方或扁平状，下方仅为薄层结缔组织和少量平滑肌，肌纤维环绕于肺泡的

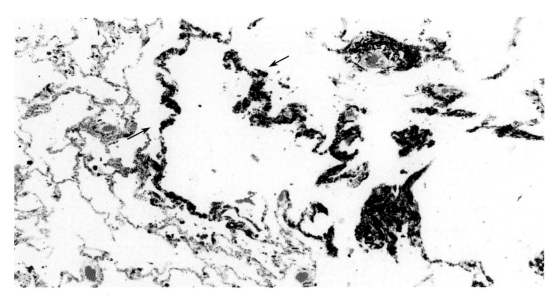

图 4　呼吸性细支气管结构(煤工尘肺):煤尘沉积在呼吸性细支气管

开口处,在纵断面的肺泡管,可见少量的平滑肌束(图 5)。

(3) 肺泡囊:是肺泡管的分支,为几个肺泡的共同的通道,结构与肺泡管相似,但在肺泡开口处无平滑肌(图 5)。

(4) 肺泡:呈多面形囊泡状,成人肺泡囊直径 200~250μm。肺脏有肺泡 3 亿 ~4 亿个。总面积可达 100m²。是肺进行气体交换的重要场所(图 5)。

肺泡壁很薄,表面衬覆上皮,上皮下肺泡间隔内有结缔组织和血管。

1) 肺泡上皮:由两种细胞组成,即Ⅰ型肺泡细胞和Ⅱ型肺泡上皮。

Ⅰ型肺泡细胞:肺泡表面大部分由Ⅰ型肺泡细胞覆盖,呈扁平状,表面光滑,核呈扁椭圆形,含核部分略厚,约 0.2μm。构成肺脏进行气体交换的广大面积。

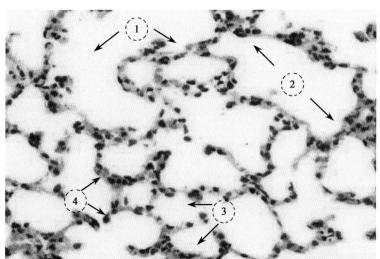

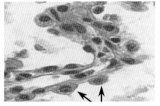

肺泡Ⅱ型上皮细胞

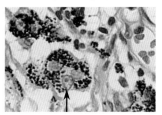

吞噬粉尘巨噬细胞

图 5　肺泡管(1)、肺泡囊(2)、肺泡(3)、肺泡隔(4)结构

Ⅱ型肺泡细胞:体积较大,呈立方形,镶嵌于Ⅰ型肺泡细胞之间。分泌表面活性物质,故又称分泌细胞。有降低肺泡表面张力、稳定肺泡直径的功能。同时,具有增生分化功能。当Ⅰ型肺泡细胞受到损伤时,Ⅱ型肺泡细胞能增生与分泌,并形成Ⅰ型肺泡细胞。起到一定的组织修复作用(图5)。

2)肺泡间隔:为相邻两个肺泡之间的薄层结缔组织。含有胶原纤维、网状纤维、弹力纤维和丰富的毛细血管网,以及成纤维细胞和巨噬细胞。肺泡间隔上有肺泡孔,使相邻肺泡相通。孔径 $10\sim15\mu m$(图5)。

3)肺泡巨噬细胞:位于肺泡间隔与肺泡腔内。体积较大,$10\sim15\mu m$,形态不一,能够伸出伪足。吞噬能力很强,胞浆内常见吞噬的物质(细菌、异物、细胞及碎片、粉尘等),具有重要的清除作用。吞噬微粒和异物的巨噬细胞,体积增大,活动性减弱,只能从气道排出(黏液 - 纤毛系统),不能再回到肺泡间隔。肺泡间隔内的这些巨噬细胞经淋巴管入淋巴结,或沉积于肺间质内(图5)。

2.2 肺间质:肺的血管、淋巴管和神经组织

2.2.1 肺的血管:肺是双重循环供血。肺动脉、肺静脉供血系统;支气管动脉、支气管静脉供血系统。

(1)肺动脉:是肺的功能血管。肺循环特点:右心室血液博出到肺动脉,肺动脉血分布于肺内毛细血管网,气体在此交换。气体交换后的毛细血管网血液回流到肺静脉,肺静脉血回流至左心房。

(2)支气管动脉:肺的营养血管。走行于各支气管的外膜中,沿途发出毛细血管,以营养各级支气管以及肺淋巴结、肺浆膜、肺血管壁和肺的结缔组织。支气管动脉分支形成的毛细血管,一部分还与肺动脉形成的毛细血管汇合,共同供血至肺泡壁。肺小叶内血液来源丰富,微循环间可有不同类型的吻合支相连接。

2.2.2 肺的淋巴管:分为两组

(1)浅组淋巴管:分布于胸膜脏层的结缔组织内,形成丰富淋巴管网,汇合成几支较大的淋巴管入肺门淋巴结。

(2)深层淋巴管:分布于支气管树的管壁内,以及肺血管周围和小叶间隔的结缔组织中。此外,在胸膜、支气管周围、血管周围、小叶间隔等处紧邻的肺泡壁上也有丰富的淋巴管,称为肺泡旁淋巴管。深部淋巴的回流,在肺门处汇合成几支淋巴管,也入肺门淋巴结。

汇入肺门淋巴结的淋巴液,经支气管 - 气管、气管旁淋巴结入右淋巴管;仅左肺上叶或其中的小部分淋巴液流入胸导管。右淋巴管与胸导管间有吻合支存在,在淋巴流压力增高时相通。

(3)淋巴管的结构

1)毛细淋巴管由一层内皮细胞组成。管壁很薄,管腔内无细胞成分。在通常切片中如不扩张,不易辨认。毛细淋巴管的基底膜或间断或缺如,内皮细胞联合处保有间隙,大分子物质易于进入。

2)集合淋巴管管壁基底膜仍有间断,内皮细胞规则,之间无细胞间隙。管壁有胶原纤维和少量平滑肌细胞。管壁内腔面有瓣膜,表面被覆连续的内皮细胞。瓣膜的作用使淋巴液只能单向流动。

2.2.3　肺的神经:来自交感神经和迷走神经分支组成的肺丛。肺丛发出分支随支气管的分支至肺组织。

(1) 迷走神经:属胆碱能纤维,神经纤维末梢分布至支气管树的平滑肌、腺体和血管。兴奋时,使支气管平滑肌收缩,而血管扩张,并刺激腺体分泌。

(2) 交感神经:属肾上腺能纤维,神经纤维末梢也分布至支气管树的平滑肌、腺体和血管。兴奋时,使支气管平滑肌松弛,而血管收缩,抑制腺体分泌。

(3) 感觉神经纤维:肺泡上皮附近、支气管黏膜、肺内结缔组织及脏层胸膜均有分布,走行于迷走神经内,以感受肺的牵张等刺激。

(孙　影　魏中秋)

煤工尘肺形态学特点

煤工尘肺(也称"煤矿尘肺")是煤矿工人在生产过程中由于长期吸入悬浮在大气中的生产性粉尘所引起尘肺病。由于产业工人所面临的生产环境不同,包括不同煤矿所处的地质条件、现场作业的不同工种、特别是吸入生产性粉尘中煤、岩尘的比例,以及是否合并有肺部感染(尤其是结核病)等因素,所引起的肺部病理变化也不尽相同。目前国内将煤工尘肺总体分为煤矽肺、矽肺和煤肺。

一般按工种划分,煤矿岩石掘进的凿岩工、装岩工等,接触的粉尘为岩石粉尘(其中游离的二氧化硅含量高达 30% 以上),所患尘肺是矽肺,如果这部分工人在长期接触岩尘后,又接触了煤尘,肺内可见煤尘沉着,可称之为矽煤肺,其本质与矽肺相同,肺内病变特点与矽肺相近。煤矿采煤工、运输工、支柱工、地面煤仓及煤场装卸工、洗煤工等接触的粉尘主要是煤尘,含游离二氧化硅浓度低于 10% 以下,如果工种未变,所患尘肺可能是煤肺。然而,在尸检材料中单纯的煤肺病例极少。而在实际工种中,煤矿工人工种多有变动,接触的粉尘是煤矽混合性粉尘,所以在我国,煤矿工人的尘肺病变多以煤矽肺最为常见。在我们收集的 47 例煤矿工人尸检标本中,绝大部分病例表现为煤矽肺的病变特点,而单纯的矽肺和煤肺的标本均比较少。

1 煤工尘肺大体形态学特点[1,3,12]

1.1 煤斑灶:包括胸膜煤斑灶和肺内煤斑灶

煤工尘肺最常见的病变就是在胸膜(脏层)和全肺内见到黑色粉尘沉积后的斑灶样病变,直径 3~5mm。根据是否形成实性病灶,这种斑灶样病变可分为煤斑和煤尘灶,这两种形态特征在全肺大切片标本中和显微镜下能被区分,但在大体标本观察时,很难用肉眼进行准确的分型,所以大体上统称为煤斑灶(coal dust maculae)。

1.1.1 胸膜煤斑灶:肺膜(脏层胸膜)表面散在分布大小不一黑色团斑,圆形或类圆形,直径 3~5mm,局部可见黑斑融合成片。触摸时,质地柔软。由于黑色煤尘沿着小叶间隔及其与肺膜连接处沉积,在肺膜表面勾画出了小叶的轮廓,因此胸膜煤斑灶边界清晰。

1.1.2　肺内煤斑灶:在肺切面上,可见与胸膜类同的黑色团斑。肺内煤斑灶多伴有小叶中心型肺气肿,呈现为圆形或类圆形的黑色囊泡状,直径 3~5mm。如果煤斑灶分布较分散,边界清晰;如果毗邻煤斑灶融合成片,病灶边界不清。肺组织表面可呈海绵状。

在肺大切片标本中,根据黑色团斑(气肿)病变有无实性病灶,这种煤斑灶可分为无明显实变病灶的"尘斑(气肿)"和有实变病灶的"尘灶(气肿)"。

往往在煤斑灶的实性病灶形成时,在肺内、胸膜下多形成黑色类圆形或星芒状实性病灶,质地较坚韧,似橡胶样。当直径超过 5mm 时,则称为煤结节。

1.2　结节病变:按病理分型可以分为矽(煤)结节和煤(矽)结节两类

在我们收集的 47 例煤矿工人尸检肺部标本中,肉眼观察结节性病灶均为黑色或灰黑色圆形、类圆形,直径多为 2~5 mm。单从大体标本上很难区分是矽(煤)结节或是煤(矽)结节。

1.2.1　煤(矽)结节(即煤矽结节):灰黑,质硬,圆形或椭圆形,一般为 3~5mm。与矽结节区别在于,具有矽(煤)结节结构的核心,周围有较厚层的"煤尘沉着带"环绕。

1.2.2　矽(煤)结节(即矽结节):灰黑,质硬,圆形或椭圆形,一般为 2~3mm(煤工尘肺典型的矽结节少见)。

1.3　块状纤维化:包括进行性块状纤维化,结节融合型块状纤维化和混合型块状纤维化

1.3.1　进行性块状纤维化:肺组织出现≥2cm×2cm×1cm 致密的一致性黑色块状病变,质地硬韧,似橡胶样。其内可见被破坏塌陷的支气管和血管。当伴有组织坏死时,可见裂隙样坏死空洞形成。

1.3.2　结节融合型块状纤维化:肺组织出现≥2cm×2cm×1cm 致密的黑色块状病变,质地硬韧。团块内可见圆形、类圆形结节样结构相互融合。

1.3.3　混合型块状纤维化:肺组织出现≥2cm×2cm×1cm 致密的黑色块状病变,质地硬韧。可见进行性块状纤维化和结节融合型块状纤维化混合的病变特点。

值得一提的是:根据形成方式,块状纤维化曾被分为进行性块状纤维化和结节融合型块状纤维化。但在我们观察的煤工尘肺尸检标本中,除可以看到上述两种类型外,还在肺内纤维化团块中见到既有结节的融合,又有进行性块状纤维化的形成。因此,在这里提出了混合型块状纤维化的分型。

1.4　弥漫性间质纤维化

煤工尘肺各种类型的病变一般都会伴有弥漫性间质纤维化,严重者肺组织呈现垂柳状、条索状外观,肺组织原有结构被损坏。

1.5　肺气肿病变

围绕在黑色煤斑灶、煤(矽)结节周围,每每可见扩张的囊泡样结构。有时囊泡破裂融合形成直径大于 1cm 的大泡型肺气肿。在大泡型肺气肿囊腔内可见悬挂在其中的条索状残存的血管与结缔组织等。

1.6 淋巴结的病变(多见肺门淋巴结的累及)

受累及的淋巴结肿大、黑色,质地硬韧,伴有钙化时,可见呈"白垩"样点状结构。严重钙化可呈"蛋壳"样外观。

1.7 胸膜病变

胸膜粘连、增厚。严重者发生玻璃样变性,甚至骨化,呈灰白色半透明状,质地硬韧、类似软骨样外观。

1.8 煤工尘肺伴发肺结核病

1.8.1 煤斑灶伴粟粒性播散性肺结核:肺内弥漫散布黑色煤斑灶,并可见灰白色粟粒状干酪样坏死遍布全肺。

1.8.2 块状纤维化伴粟粒性播散性肺结核:左肺上叶接近叶间裂处可见黑色纤维斑块,斑块内有数个白色斑点(干酪样坏死结核病灶)。左肺上叶灰白色弥漫性变实,油腻干酪状外观,下叶密布粟粒性结核播散病灶(见图谱部分图31、图32)。

1.8.3 煤工尘肺伴肺门淋巴结结核病变:肺门淋巴结肿大,可见灰黑色粉尘沉积,其间夹杂灰白色干酪样坏死病变。

1.9 煤工尘肺伴发肺癌

1.9.1 煤工尘肺伴结节型肺癌:煤工尘肺肺组织中可见圆形、类圆形瘤样结节,灰白或灰黄色、质地较细腻、松软。

1.9.2 煤工尘肺伴弥漫型肺癌:煤尘沉积的肺组织内弥漫遍布大小不等灰黄色的瘤样结节。

1.10 煤工尘肺伴发肺源性心脏病

煤工尘肺时,可因肺部一些慢性疾病而引起肺循环阻力增加,肺动脉压力持续升高而导致的以右心室肥厚、心室腔扩张为特征的心脏病。此时,心脏体积增大,重量增加,肺动脉圆锥膨隆,心尖圆顿。右心室肥厚,心室腔扩张。右心室肉柱及乳头肌增粗。右心室前壁增厚。

(徐 洪 刘和亮)

2 煤工尘肺组织形态学特点[1-12]

2.1 煤矽肺

2.1.1 煤斑(coal dust dots,区别于大体的煤斑灶 coal dust maculae):包括胸膜煤斑和肺内煤斑。

(1)胸膜煤斑:胸膜面的黑斑或黑色条纹,位于胸膜内、胸膜下或胸膜与小叶间隔连接处。镜下为大量吞噬煤尘的巨噬细胞(煤尘细胞)聚集而成。煤尘细胞间有网状纤维或少量胶原纤维增生。

（2）肺内煤斑：由沉着在细、小支气管和小血管周围，以及呼吸性细支气管所属的呼吸道的煤尘细胞构成。此处尚无较大的实性、灶状病变形成。每每伴有小叶中心型肺气肿。这可能是煤矿尘肺的一种比较特殊的病理类型。

2.1.2 煤尘灶：较多的煤尘细胞沉着在细、小支气管和小血管周围，以及呼吸性细支气管所属的呼吸道。由于吞噬了煤尘颗粒的巨噬细胞具有较强的游走能力，因此煤尘细胞沿着肺泡道、肺泡壁伸延，并扩展到邻近的肺泡。当较多的煤尘聚集时，阻塞小气道形成肺气肿。

典型病变为巨噬细胞和／或增生的纤维组织构成中心部的实性病灶，伴肺气肿形成。与煤斑气肿的区别就是在病变中心部形成灶状结构为实性的。灶状结构可呈现出各式各样的形态，如：星芒状、蟹足状、海星状、游鱼状、骡马状、飞禽状等等。根据增生纤维组织成分的差异分为两种类型，即煤尘细胞灶和煤尘纤维灶。

（1）煤尘细胞灶：主要由煤尘细胞聚集而成，形成各种形状的黑色实变灶，伴阻塞性肺气肿形成。此时病灶中胶原纤维成分较少，镀银染色，病灶中可见网状纤维。

（2）煤尘纤维灶：大量煤尘细胞聚集形成各种形状的实变灶，病灶中胶原纤维成分增多（但不超过组成成分的 50%），走行方向不一，伴阻塞性肺气肿形成。

2.1.3 结节病变：为圆形、类圆形结节样结构。根据病变演变过程，可以大致分为细胞性结节、细胞纤维性结节和纤维性结节。

（1）巨噬细胞性肺泡炎：任何外源性刺激物，如粉尘、化学性、物理性、生物性致敏原等进入并潴留在肺泡时，首先引起巨噬细胞性肺泡炎。

初始病变为大量浸润的中性粒细胞为主的炎性物质充填在肺泡内。随后巨噬细胞增多并逐渐取代中性粒细胞，最终表现为大量巨噬细胞充填在肺泡腔内，其间夹杂一些中性粒细胞、脱落的上皮细胞和其他脂类、蛋白类的成分，形成所谓的巨噬细胞性肺泡炎。当巨噬细胞吞噬了煤尘颗粒后，巨噬细胞胞体增大，胞浆内含有黑色的煤尘颗粒。吞噬煤尘颗粒的巨噬细胞大量聚集在肺泡腔内，逐渐形成结节状肉芽肿样结构，过渡到细胞性结节病变。

（2）细胞性结节：主要由吞噬煤尘的巨噬细胞聚集形成圆形、类圆形的结节样结构（煤尘细胞性肉芽肿结构），细胞间仅见少量增生的胶原。

（3）细胞纤维性结节：在吞噬煤尘的巨噬细胞间，成纤维细胞增生伴较多胶原纤维沉积。

（4）纤维性结节：除大量沉积的煤尘细胞外，胶原增生显著，呈条索、纤维状分布。典型者中央为呈同心圆状增生的胶原纤维，有时胶原纤维可发生玻璃样变性，由煤尘细胞聚集形成的较厚的"套袖样"结构环绕在结节外围，并伸出"伪足"向周围间质呈放射状伸延，病理学称之为煤矽结节。

值得一提的是：①煤矽结节与后面提及的矽（煤）结节（即矽结节）主要区别是：煤矽结节具有的类似于矽结节结构的核心较小，期间煤尘沉着较多，周围有较厚的"套袖"状煤尘沉着带（一般超过结节面积的 1/3）或放射状伪足样结构向周围间质伸延。②煤工尘肺中，有些实性病变（尤其是直径超过 5mm）介于煤尘纤维灶与结节性病变之间。即病灶内增生的胶原纤维超过了组成成分的 50%，而镜下结构则呈现出明显的星芒状、多角形或不规则形，胶原束走行方向不定，煤尘细胞分散在胶原束之间。增生的纤维组织常沿着间质向周围呈伪足状伸延。有学者将其归为一种相对独立的病变，称之为交界性煤尘纤维灶或非典型煤矽结节。

2.1.4 煤尘性块状纤维化:是煤矽肺Ⅲ期的表现。肺组织出现≥2cm×2cm×1cm团块状结构,期间可伴有浓集的煤尘及塌陷崩解的肺组织碎片,可见坏死性煤尘性空洞形成。分为进行性块状纤维化、结节融合型块状纤维化和混合型块状纤维化。

(1)进行性块状纤维化:主要由弥漫增生的胶原纤维夹杂大量沉积的煤尘构成,其间多见煤尘密集沉积形成黑色"煤尘池"以及坏死性"煤尘性空洞"。

(2)结节融合型块状纤维化:为密集融合的煤矽结节形成的团块状病变,其间夹杂煤尘细胞。

(3)混合型块状纤维化:可见上述两种结构混杂在一起构成。

2.1.5 煤尘性间质纤维化:煤矿粉尘和煤尘细胞沉着在胸膜、小叶间隔、肺泡道、细小支气管和小血管周围,出现间质成纤维细胞增生及数量不等的纤维组织增生,形成弥漫性纤维网络,损坏肺组织的原有结构。在煤矽肺病变,除灶状、结节性病变外,煤尘性间质纤维化病变占有重要地位。一般讲,凡有煤尘沉着,就伴有间质纤维化。间质纤维化形成时,间质内有时还可见平滑肌组织增生。

煤尘性间质纤维化常起自呼吸性细支气管,并向肺泡间隔、小叶间隔发展,同时可向细小支气管及小血管周围蔓延。有时,增生的纤维组织像"蟹足样"伸延到周围组织中。除肺间质纤维组织增生外,波及小叶间隔时,小叶间隔明显增宽,波及胸膜时,胸膜及其胸膜下纤维组织增生致使胸膜增厚,其间夹杂煤尘沉着。由于有黑色煤尘夹杂在增生的纤维化组织中,所以煤工尘肺间质纤维化部分呈现黑色外观,这可能是有别于其他金属矿山尘肺的间质纤维化。

(杨 方 孙 影)

2.2 矽煤肺(矽肺)

2.2.1 巨噬细胞性肺泡炎:基本病变同上述的煤矽肺时的巨噬细胞肺泡炎。但由于,是含游离的矽尘颗粒引起的病变,因此吞噬矽尘的巨噬细胞一般不呈现黑褐色的外观。

2.2.2 矽(煤)结节(又称矽结节):结节大小在 0.2~1.5mm。典型的结节,在 H.E 染色时,增生的胶原纤维呈同心圆样,中心区的胶原有时发生玻璃样变,表现为均匀红染,Masson三色染色时,增生的胶原纤维染成蓝色,天狼星红染色(偏振光显微镜下观察)可见结节内绿色Ⅲ型胶原与红橙色Ⅰ型胶原交织在一起。在结节内和/或结节外有数量不等的煤尘沉着。

应该说,在煤矿工人尘肺病变中,肺内典型的矽结节是比较少见的。一般我们只是从煤尘细胞是否形成比较明显的"套袖样"结构,并围绕在结节的外周来确定是矽结节还是煤矽结节。显然,形态学很难十分明确地将这两者截然分开。在这里,为了理解方便,我们做一界定:如果结节外围煤尘细胞形成的"套袖样"结构或伪足样结构超过结节面积1/3,为煤矽结节,如果煤尘细胞形成的外套较薄(小于结节面积1/3)或不完整,为矽结节。

与肺组织相比较,淋巴结质地较实,因此当累及的淋巴结内发生结节病变时,有时可见相对比较典型的矽结节形成。

2.2.3 矽肺块状纤维化:由矽结节病变继续发展而来,多由肺内矽结节的密集融合而成。镜下可见多数玻璃样变性的矽结节紧密靠拢、互相融合,但矽结节的轮廓多可辨认。有时矽结节排列稀疏,结节间为大量增生的结缔组织与沉积的煤尘。有时在融合的结节内可见细小支气管、小血管及萎陷的肺泡等。

矽煤肺病变的块状纤维化,很少有进行性块状纤维化,一般多由结节融合发展形成。因此病灶以矽结节融合为主,伴有数量不等的纤维组织的增生。这也与煤矽肺在块状纤维化形成方式与类型分型中有所不同。

2.2.4 尘性间质纤维化:基本病变同煤矽肺。但由于矽尘颗粒更为硬韧,因此所致纤维化范围与程度较煤矽肺更加严重。

2.3 煤肺

单纯的煤尘,因为所含二氧化硅量极低,是否能导致肺部特异性病变,长期以来存在着分歧与争议。因此,针对煤尘沉积所致的病变,临床上很少对单纯煤肺进行诊断。

然而,较多形态学发现,吸入含矽量低的煤尘,在肺及其引流的淋巴组织内可形成相应病变,即如前所述的煤斑、煤尘灶、灶旁肺气肿、煤尘性间质纤维化等病变。而不存在典型的结节样病变,即没有矽结节和煤矽结节的形成。镜下观察为,前述的肺内煤斑、煤尘灶和小叶中心型肺气肿,可伴有不同程度的间质纤维化形成(肉眼,胸膜表面有大量黑斑,每有相互的融合。切面上肺内出现煤斑灶、小叶中心型肺气肿。有时煤尘沉积较多时,肺实质变成乌黑色)。淋巴结内大量煤尘细胞沉积,有处可见轻度的间质纤维化形成(肉眼累及的淋巴结为黑色、略大,但质地较软,不融合)。

(刘和亮　徐　洪)

2.4 伴发性病变

2.4.1 合并肺结核病[21-24]:煤工尘肺病变越重,肺结核病发率越高,Ⅲ期矽肺患者并发率可高达75%。使原有的煤工尘肺病变更复杂,更严重。患者肺内可形成空洞或侵及大血管致肺内大出血而死亡。根据病理特点,分为结合型与分离型。

(1)分离型:为煤工尘肺病变和结核病变并存,并保持各自的病变特征,如煤工尘肺结节性病变与结核病的结节性病变显示各自的形态结构特点,典型者既有煤矽结节形成,也有结核结节形成。

(2)结合型:则为煤工尘肺病变和结核病变互相结合,融为一体,失去各自病变特点,典型者形成煤矽结核结节。

煤矽结核结节较大,周围有较厚的纤维层包绕,纤维层内及其周边有较多煤尘沉着。结节中心部则是大片干酪样坏死,中央或一侧有时可见变性、坏死的煤矽结节,其间有数量不等的吞噬煤尘的巨噬细胞和游离的煤尘颗粒。多数煤矽结核结节内,仅见干酪样坏死物,而不见上皮样细胞增生、郎罕氏巨细胞形成及淋巴细胞浸润。但有些结节内有干酪样坏死的同时,也有少量上皮样细胞、或不典型的多核巨细胞和淋巴细胞。

有时,在煤矽结核结节边缘伴渗出性结核病变或增殖性病变,可能经过融合、坏死及纤维包裹而形成煤矽结核结节。严重病例,多数煤矽结核结节融合,或煤矽结核结节、结核结节、煤矽结节及其尘性病变或结核病变相互融合形成团块,且容易形成空洞。

有时结核病变出现在支气管,表现为尘性支气管炎基础上伴随有干酪样坏死等病变,称之为尘性结核性支气管炎。

煤工尘肺合并结核时,肺内还可见其他反应形式的结核性病变和煤矽肺的病变,使其在形态上颇为复杂多样。

2.4.2　合并肺肿瘤[25-29]：矿物粉尘起着类似致癌物的作用。因此在煤工尘肺病例中可见各种类型的肺癌(如小细胞肺癌和非小细胞肺癌,包括肺腺癌、肺鳞癌、肺腺鳞癌等)和其他恶性肿瘤(如恶性间皮瘤)的发生。

2.5　其他病变

矿山粉尘(包括煤工尘肺粉尘)具有较强的"侵袭"性,由呼吸道进入体内后,经淋巴循环运载并与清除。当粉尘在淋巴结内大量沉积后,除破坏淋巴结组织、诱发淋巴结纤维化外,还可突破淋巴结被膜侵入邻近组织与器官,破坏组织结构并造成功能障碍。在我们47例煤工尘肺尸检标本中,常累及的组织与器官如下。

2.5.1　淋巴结的病变：煤尘进入呼吸道,经淋巴系统清除。吸入到肺内的煤尘经肺的浅层、深层的淋巴结转送,在胸膜、肺内支气管和血管周围淋巴组织内特别是在肺门淋巴结、穿隆下淋巴结和气管旁淋巴结等沉积,形成淋巴结内病变。根据病变进展情况,分为淋巴结内煤尘沉着、淋巴结内纤维组织增生、纤维化和淋巴结内结节病变形成。

(1)淋巴结内煤尘沉着：首先煤尘细胞集聚在髓窦内,随着尘细胞的增多,局部淋巴结结构消失,被吞噬黑色煤尘的巨噬细胞所代替,并可累及皮质。煤尘细胞间网状纤维增多。

(2)淋巴结内纤维组织增生：淋巴结内伴随着煤尘沉积,出现成纤维细胞和结缔组织增生,纤维化区域淋巴结结构破坏消失。

(3)结节病变形成：在煤尘沉着和纤维化的背景上,出现结节结构,包括细胞性结节、细胞纤维性结节和纤维性结节(可见煤矽结节与矽结节形成)。

(4)煤工尘肺合并结核时,病变易累及到淋巴结(最常见为肺门淋巴结、支气管旁淋巴结),除煤尘沉积在淋巴结造成的病变(如:煤矽结节、间质纤维化等)外,合并有结核所致的病变,典型者就是煤矽结核结节形成。有时结节相互融合,在淋巴结内形成巨大的融合性结节,原有结构被完全破坏。

2.5.2　支气管的累及与病变：最易受累及的支气管是靠近肺门淋巴结的总支气管和叶支气管。表现为,支气管壁不同程度被侵入的纤维化组织破坏,严重时可累及支气管全层。具有侵袭性增生的纤维化组织主要包括成纤维细胞(包括肌成纤维细胞),一定数量的胶原纤维,及其夹杂其间的大量尘细胞。增生的纤维化组织由支气管外膜向黏膜侵入,侵入黏膜时,增生的纤维化组织可呈息肉状突入支气管腔,侵入黏膜下层时,纤维化组织可分割腺泡或导管,致腺体萎缩,增生的纤维化组织还可突破壁内软骨膜,破坏软骨细胞。有时支气管壁可见结节性病灶形成。

值得提出的是,煤矿尘肺时,往往伴发支气管炎性病变,在此基础上若伴有煤尘细胞侵犯,称为"尘性支气管炎"。支气管壁黏液腺肥大、增生,黏膜上皮杯状细胞增多,黏液分泌亢进,各级支气管腔内有黏液炎性分泌物储留。有时黏膜上皮可见鳞状上皮化生。支气管各层,尤其是黏膜下层有数量不等的炎细胞浸润(以淋巴细胞浸润为主),在炎细胞间夹杂吞噬煤尘的巨噬细胞。当间质纤维化波及管壁,可破坏管壁结构。各级支气管壁外膜有煤尘细胞沉积,以呼吸性支气管壁煤尘细胞沉积最为显著。

值得强调的是,"尘性支气管炎"往往是在支气管慢性炎症的基础上形成的。此时,支气管壁已有纤维组织增生。因此,我们很难判断煤尘沉积与炎症病变在促进支气管壁及其间质纤维化方面的"主、次"作用。

2.5.3　胸膜的累及与病变:进入肺内邻近胸膜肺实质的煤尘,经淋巴引流首先到达胸膜并沉积,伴胸膜下方小血管扩张充血、增生;纤维组织增生、致使胸膜增厚、粘连;每每可见,沉积在胸膜之下的黑色煤尘沿着小叶间隔伸延侵入,将小叶轮廓勾画的十分清晰,形成胸膜及胸膜下煤斑灶,有时在增厚的胸膜内偶有煤矽结节及增生的血管内血栓形成,在胸膜的纤维化病变中可见组织的坏死与钙化。

2.5.4　煤尘性肺气肿:进入到肺内的煤尘,可以沉积在肺内支气管及其各级分支,导致管壁增厚,甚至管腔狭窄。特别是煤尘沉积于终末细支气管及其远端部分(呼吸性细支气管、肺泡管、肺泡囊和肺泡等部分),可致小气道扩张并伴有肺泡壁的破坏,形成肺气肿病变。

肺内煤斑或煤尘灶的周围,每有扩张的小气腔,居于肺小叶的中心,称之为小叶中央型肺气肿。煤工尘肺时,最常见的是煤斑伴肺气肿形成和煤尘灶伴肺气肿的形成。严重病例,肺气肿扩展到多数肺泡囊及肺泡道,则可形成全小叶破坏型肺气肿。病变区为 1cm 左右的黑色囊状气腔,腔内可见残留的小血管及间质结构形成"架桥"状间隔,进一步发展可形成大泡型肺气肿。

2.5.5　小血管的累及与病变:煤尘沉积在肺内动、静脉及其分支。纤维化的组织由外向内侵入肺动脉壁外膜和中膜,可见弹力纤维断裂,结构的破坏伴有煤尘的沉积。肺静脉壁薄,纤维化病变可侵入静脉全层,致静脉内膜不平,静脉全层受累"黑染"。一些煤尘病灶或结节中央每每见到受累及的小血管被裹挟其中,有时伴血栓形成。高倍镜下,可见煤尘"突破"小血管壁,进入血管腔内,与腔内的血细胞混杂在一起。

2.5.6　脂肪组织的累及:煤尘沉积伴间质纤维化病变还可累及到支气管外膜的脂肪组织,可见脂肪组织中大量尘细胞聚集,并伴有脂肪组织中细小血管的增生、扩张、充血等病理变化。

2.5.7　淋巴管的累及:肺内各级淋巴管的回流是清除肺内煤尘的主要途径之一。当大量煤尘进入肺内,可导致肺内淋巴管开放与扩张,每每可见扩张的淋巴管内充满黑色的煤尘,淋巴管壁增厚。

2.5.8　神经纤维的累及:当煤尘沉积在肺内或支气管壁时,可向周围组织侵袭,累及肺组织内或支气管壁内或壁周的神经干和神经节。此时可见煤尘侵破神经束外膜进入神经干。

2.5.9　肺内继发各种感染性病变:由于煤尘进入呼吸道,致机体抵抗力降低,肺内可继发细菌、病毒及其他病原菌感染,导致肺内发生各种感染性病变(如化脓性炎、浆液性炎、纤维素炎或混合性炎及其脓肿形成等)。

2.5.10　棒状小体(含铁小体)[9]:在 47 例煤工尘肺尸检病例中,有较多病例的肺组织中均可发现棒状小体的形成。光镜下小体大小不一,长度多为 15~50μm。小体形似棒状、纤维桩、哑铃状、串珠状。多有一黑色或透明折光性较强的轴心。多分布与肺泡腔、肺泡壁,可裹挟于沉积在肺内的煤尘中,可呈簇出现,也可游离于肺泡腔内。在煤工尘肺病变中,如煤尘灶、煤矽结节及其间质纤维化区域内有时也可有棒状小体的存在。有关棒状小体与煤工尘肺发病学的关系,报道较少,李洪珍等认为这种小体与石棉肺中石棉小体相似。又因为小体含有铁蛋白成分,称之为"含铁小体",可能与尘肺发生时的巨噬细胞聚集、肺泡Ⅱ型上皮细胞增生及其间质纤维化的形成有一定的关联。

2.5.11　肌成纤维细胞分化[33-36]:在长期受到致纤维化因素的刺激时,肺支气管黏膜上皮细胞和间质成纤维细胞,将会发生表型转变并分化成为"肌成纤维细胞",特异性表达平滑肌肌动蛋白。肺支气管黏膜上皮细胞和间质成纤维细胞向肌成纤维细胞的分化在肺纤维化的发生与发展过程中起着关键性作用。煤工尘肺病变标本中,我们发现,在结节病变与间质纤维化病变中,均有平滑肌肌动蛋白阳性表达的肌成纤维细胞的存在。在动物模型标本中,证实了这些肌成纤维细胞来源于肺间质的成纤维细胞和肺泡Ⅱ型上皮细胞。初步揭示尘肺纤维化病变中肌成纤维细胞转化的细胞来源和作用。

2.5.12 肺源性心脏病:在47例煤工尘肺尸检标本中,有肺脏和心脏标本的共21例,其中伴发右心室肥厚、扩张的有9例。镜下可见,右心室心肌纤维增粗、核大深染,呈不规则形。右室心肌组织可发生局灶状坏死或纤维化、瘢痕化。伴心肌间质水肿和胶原纤维增生。

此外,有时可见煤尘经病变处的血管进入血流,在肝脏、脾脏等器官沉积。

(宋旭东　魏中秋　杨　方)

参考文献

［1］李洪珍,李铁生.120例煤矿工人肺部病理变化与煤矽肺病理诊断的关系[J].职业卫生与病伤,1989,4(1):1-4.

［2］李铁生,李洪珍.间质硬化型矽肺的病理观察[J].中国综合临床,1980,1:30-35.

［3］李洪珍,李铁生.煤矿尘肺的病理类型[J].煤矿医学,1982,4(增刊):72-74.

［4］李洪珍,李铁生.煤矿尘肺病理形态标准[J].煤矿医学,1982,4(增刊):69-71.

［5］李洪珍,李铁生.煤矿尘肺基本的病理变化[J].煤矿医学,1982,4(增刊):65-68.

［6］李铁生,李洪珍.煤矿工人尘肺结节性病变的观察[J].煤矿医学,1981,3(2):1-4.

［7］李洪珍,李铁生.生产性粉尘在肺内沉着[J].煤矿医学,1981,3(3):31-35.

［8］李铁生,李洪珍.煤矿尘肺肺部并发症对病变的影响[J].煤矿医学,1982,4(增刊):75-77.

［9］李洪珍,王洪原,孟韶阁,等.煤矿尘肺含铁小体的形态及尘肺病变特点观察[J].中华病理杂志,1991,20(3):169-171.

［10］李洪珍,李铁生.煤尘及煤矽混合性粉尘所致大白鼠肺脏的形态学变化[J].职业卫生与病伤,1989,4(3):7-12.

［11］王献华,李铁生,杨方,等.咽泰对大鼠慢性染煤尘的实验性煤肺病变疗效的观察[J].中国煤炭工业医学杂志,1998,5(1):477-479.

［12］李洪珍,李铁生.煤矿尘肺病理组织学图谱[M].北京:能源出版社,1987.

［13］戴宇飞,秦立强,张作文.2010—2017年职业卫生与职业病领域国家自然科学基金资助项目分析[J].中华预防医学杂志,2018,52(7):769-771.

［14］Bing Han,Hongbo Liu,Guojiang Zhai,et al.Estimates and Predictions of Coal Workers' Pneumoconiosis Cases among Redeployed Coal Workers of the Fuxin Mining Industry Group in China:A Historical Cohort Study[J].PLoS One,2016,11(2):e0148179.

［15］Cheng BW,Su M. International incidence trend of coal workers' pneumoconiosis[J].中华劳动卫生职业病杂志,2019,37(1):75-78.

［16］Han S,Chen H,Harvey MA,et al. Focusing on Coal Workers' Lung Diseases:A Comparative Analysis of China,Australia,and the United States[J].Int J Environ Res Public Health,2018,15(11).:E2565.

［17］中国煤炭工业协会.2017煤炭行业发展年度报告,2018-3-27.

［18］国家统计局.第三次全国经济普查,2016-3-1.

［19］李德鸿.不要把尘肺病防治引入歧途[J].环境与职业医学,2018,35(4):283-285.

［20］中华人民共和国国家卫生健康委员会.http://www.nhc.gov.cn/guihuaxxs/ s10748/201905/9b8d52727cf346049de8acce25ffcbd0.shtml.

［21］孟韶阁,等.矿山矽肺与结核防治［M］.北京:能源出版社,1985.

［22］杨方.尘肺肺结核的病理［M］//钟明,等.尘肺合并症.北京:中国医药科技出版社,1993,45-48.

［23］Yew WW,Leung CC,Chang KC,et al. Can treatment outcomes of latent TB infection and TB in silicosis be improved?［J］.J Thorac Dis,2019,11(1):E8-E10.

［24］Skowroński M1,Halicka A,Barinow-Wojewódzki A. Pulmonary tuberculosis in a male with silicosis［J］. Adv Respir Med,2018,86(3). doi:10.5603.24.

［25］王光华.煤工尘肺合并肺癌 31 例诊治体会［J］.实用医技杂志,2010,17(3):258-259.

［26］包树文.煤工尘肺合并肺癌 38 例分析［J］.吉林医学,2012,33(18):3972.

［27］Manno M,Levy L,Johanson G,et al. silicosis and lung cancer:what level of exposure is acceptable?［J］. Med Lav,2018;109(6):478-480.

［28］Sato T,Shimosato T,Klinman DM. Silicosis and lung cancer:current perspectives［J］. Lung Cancer, 2018,9:91-101.

［29］Mlika M,Adigun R. Silicosis (Coal Worker Pneumoconiosis). Source stat pearls［Internet］. Treasure Island(FL):StatPearls Publishing,2019.

［30］赵培真,杨方.中国年轻人动脉粥样硬化病理生物学图谱［M］.北京:中国协和医科大学出版社,2006.

［31］徐洪,杨方,袁媛,等.免疫组织化学 Image Pro Plus 图像半定量分析的参数选择［J］.解剖学杂志, 2012,35(1):37-41.

［32］杨方,赵培真,佘铭鹏,等.人冠状动脉几种细胞外基质的动态变化与动脉粥样硬化形成的关系［J］. 中华病理学杂志,1998,27(3):177-181.

［33］Bonan Zhang,Hong Xu,Yi Zhang,et al. Targeting the RAS axis alleviates silicotic fibrosis and Ang Ⅱ-inducedmyofibroblast differentiation via inhibition of the hedgehog signalingpathway［J］. Toxicology Letters,2019,313:30-41.

［34］张惠,徐丁洁,毛娜,等.乙酰化微管蛋白在矽肺成纤维细胞中定位及表达变化［J］.中国职业医学, 2018,45(2):150-156.

［35］Deng H,Xu H,Zhang X,et al. Protective effect of Ac-SDKP on alveolar epithelial cells through inhibition of EMT via TGF-β1/ROCK1 pathway in silicosis in rat［J］. Toxicol Appl Pharmacol,2016,16(294):1-10.

［36］Li Shifeng,Xu Hong,Yi Xue,et al. Ac-SDKP increases α-TAT 1 and promotes the apoptosis in lung fibroblasts and epithelial cells double-stimulated with TGF-β1 and silica［J］. Toxicology and Applied Pharmacology,2019,369:17-29.

［37］苏敏、邹昌琪.尘肺病理诊断图谱［M］.北京:人民卫生出版社,2019.

［38］邹仲之,李继承.组织学与胚胎学［J］.北京:人民卫生出版社,2013.

［39］柏树令,应大君.系解剖学［J］.北京:人民卫生出版社,2013.

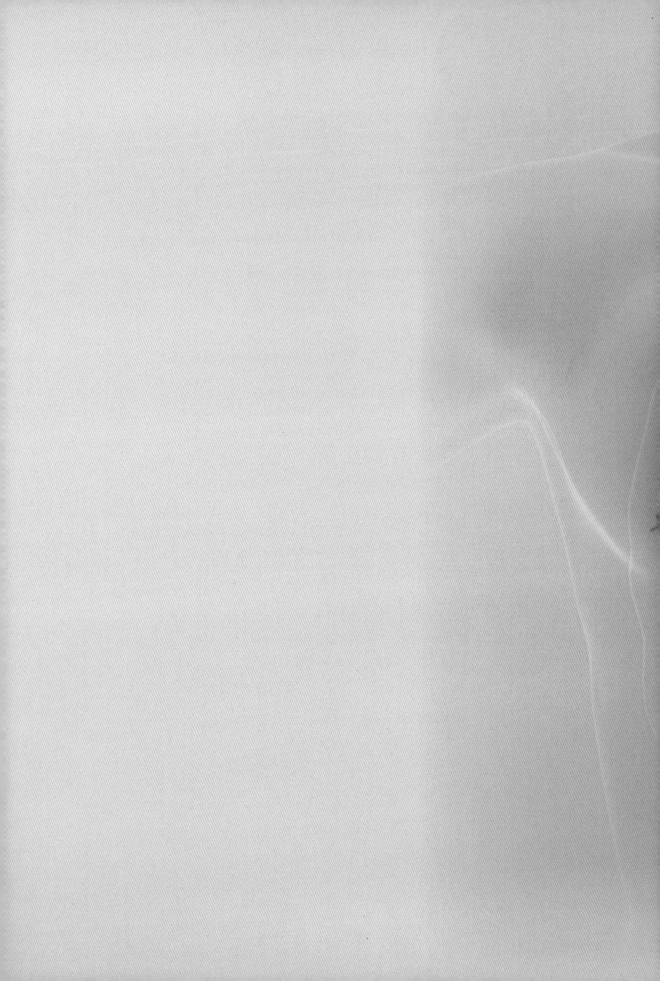

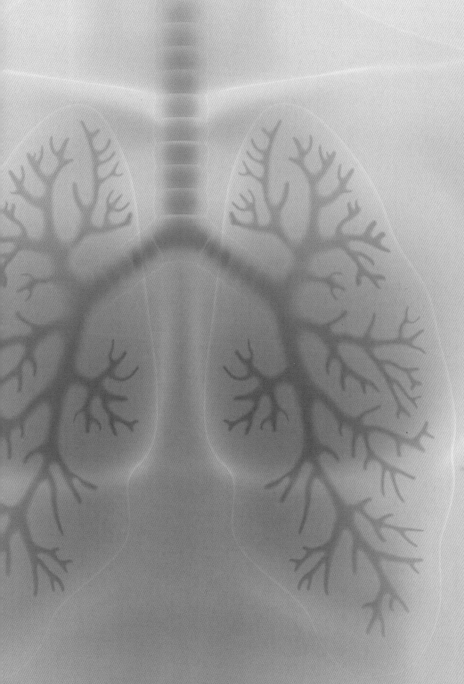

Atlas Guide

Part I

Anatomy and Histology of Lung[38,39]

1 Anatomy of the lung

The lungs locate at thorax, the left and the right lung standing at the sides of mediastinum and above the diaphragm. The left lung is divided into two lobes (upper and lower) separated by an oblique fissure, and the right one is divided into three lobes (upper, middle and lower) separated by a horizontal fissure and oblique fissure (Fig.1).

Trachea and bronchi, composed of cartilage, muscle, mucosa and connective tissue, are bridge to connect the left lung with the right one. On entering the hilum of the lung, each main (primary) bronchus divides into lobar bronchi (secondary bronchi), and each lobar bronchus

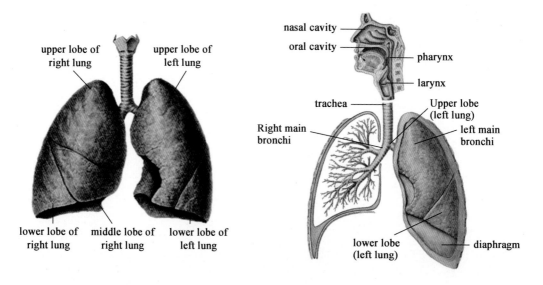

Fig. 1　Anatomy of the lung

gives rise to segmental bronchi (third bronchi). The segmental bronchi branch repeatedly, finally creating the bronchial tree.

Trachea usually branches for 25 times and finally gives rise to alveoli. The segmental bronchi (third bronchi) correspond the pyramid-shaped bronchopulmonary segments, whose tips terminate pulmonary hilum. Bronchopulmonary segments are separated by thin connective tissue, being the independent structural and functional units of lungs.

Bronchopulmonary segment is divided into pulmonary lobules, being the grossly visible minimum units. Pulmonary lobules are normally less than 1 cm in diameter. The tips of pyramid-shaped pulmonary lobules are the entrances for the bronchioli, blood vessels and lymphatic vessels. Pulmonary lobules are well demarcated by the surrounding delicate connective tissue.

2   Histology of the lung

The lung contains parenchyma that is the branches of bronchi and alveoli and mesenchyme composed of connective tissue, blood vessels, lymphatic vessels and nerves.

2.1   Parenchyma：It includes conduction portion and respiratory portion.

2.1.1   Conduction portion：This portion conducts air into the lung. Each main bronchus branches into lobar bronchi, which are subdivided into the segmental bronchi. The branches of segmental bronchi are defined as small bronchi. Bronchioles are air-conducting ducts that measure 1 mm or less in diameter. The larger bronchioles represent branches of the small bronchi. These ducts branch repeatedly and give rise to the terminal bronchioles that is about 0.5mm in diameter. So the conduction portion consists of the bronchi, bronchioles and terminal bronchioles.

Branching of bronchi causes the decrease in bronchi diameters and wall thickness, with variation in wall structure.

（1）Bronchi and small bronchi (Fig. 2)

1）Mucosa：Mucosa is composed of epithelium and lamina propria.

Epithelium：It is lined with ciliated pseudostratified epithelium with goblet cells.

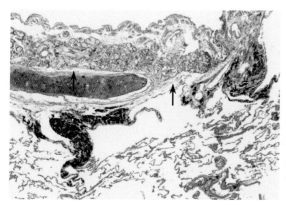 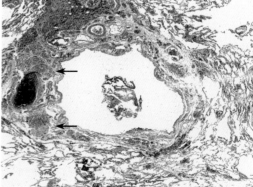

Fig. 2   Small bronchi: Mucous gland proliferation (arrows) in lung with coal workers' pneumoconiosis

Lamina propria: Located beneath the epithelium is lamina propria, appears as a typical connective tissue containing minimal collagen and numerous elastic fibers. Muscularis marks the boundary between the mucosa and submucosa.

2) Submucosa: Submucosa remains as a relatively loose connective tissue. The mixed glands are present that could secrete mucus and serous fluid.

3) Adventitia: Adventitia is moderately dense connective tissue and hyaline cartilage plates. The blood vessels, lymphatic vessels and nerves are also visible.

(2) Bronchioles (Fig. 3)

1) Mucosa

Epithelium: Epithelium is lined with a ciliated, pseudostratified or simple columnar epithelium with minimal goblet cells.

Lamina propria: A relatively increase in smooth muscle cells is present in the thinner wall of bronchioles, but still showing a discontinuous ring.

2) Submucosa: Submucosa is thin, with or without glands.

3) Adventitia: The larger-diameter bronchioles have hyaline cartilage plates that become smaller and smaller, finally disappears as branching of bronchioles. The blood vessels, lymphatic vessels and nerves are visible.

(3) Terminal bronchioles (Fig. 3)

1) Mucosa

Epithelium: It is lined with simple ciliated columnar epithelium, no goblet cells.

Lamina propria: Rings of proliferated smooth muscle cells is characteristic.

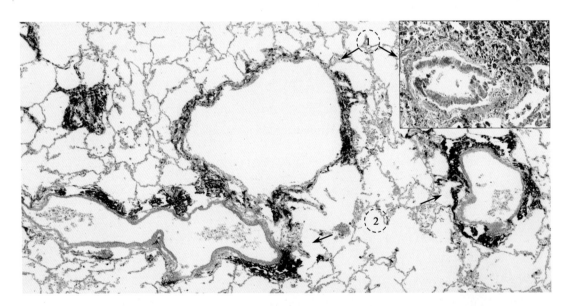

Fig. 3   Coal dust deposits in bronchioles and terminal bronchioles

1. Bronchioles: No rings of proliferated smooth muscle cells in lamina propria; 2. Terminal bronchioles: Rings of proliferated smooth muscle cells in lamina propria

2) Submucosa:Glands are absent in the thin layer of submucosa.

3) Adventitia:Adventitia has no hyaline cartilage plates,but keeping minimal blood vessels,lymphatic vessels and nerves.

2.1.2   Respiratory portion:It consists of respiratory bronchioles,alveolar ducts,alveolar sacs,and alveoli.

(1) Respiratory bronchioles:Each terminal bronchiole finally gives rise to more than 2 branches of respiratory bronchioles.(Fig. 4)

1) Epithelium:A simple ciliated columnar epithelium is present at the junction of the terminal bronchiole and respiratory bronchioles,gradually transforming into simple columnar epithelium,simple cuboidal epithelium,and simple squamous epithelium at the point of adjacent avleoli.

2) Lamina propria:The thin lamina propria contains minimal connective tissue and smooth muscle cells. Respiratory bronchioles are the first part of the bronchial tree that allows gas exchange,because scattered,thin-walled alveoli extend from the lumen of the respiratory bronchioles.

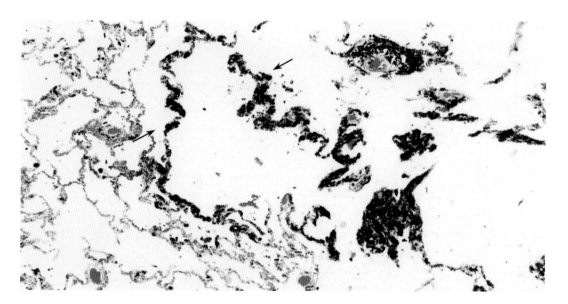

Fig. 4   Respiratory bronchioles: Coal dust deposits in the respiratory bronchioles

(2) Alveolar ducts:Respiratory bronchioles branch repeatedly for three times,transforming into the alveolar ducts. The thin wall of alveolar ducts is lined by simple cuboidal epithelium or simple squamous epithelium,and minimal connective tissue and smooth muscle cells locate beneath the epithelium. There are dense openings of alveoli in the wall of alveolar ducts,at which rings of smooth muscle(in cross section) or bands of smooth muscle(in longitudinal section)are present.(Fig. 5)

(3) Alveolar sacs: Alveolar sacs usually occur at the termination of an alveolar duct. Alveolar sacs are spaces surrounded by clusters of alveoli. The surrounding alveoli open into these spaces. The structure of alveolar sacs is similar as alveolar ducts, except no smooth muscle cells at the opening of alveoli. (Fig. 5)

(4) Alveoli: Each alveolus is a thin-walled polyhedral chamber approximately 200-250μm in diameter. About 300 to 400 million alveoli are found in adult lung; their combined internal surface area is approximately 100m^2, being the actual site of gas exchange. (Fig. 5)

The thin-walled alveolus is lined by its epithelium, which is surrounded by a network of capillaries and connective tissue.

1) Alveolar epithelium: It is composed of type Ⅰ and Ⅱ alveolar cells.

Type Ⅰ alveolar cells: Type Ⅰ alveolar cells line most of the surface of the alveoli and the sites of the gas exchange. They are simple squamous cells with smooth surface, extremely thin, a little thicker (about 0.2μm) only at the nucleus.

Type Ⅱ alveolar cells: Type Ⅱ alveolar cells with cuboidal shape, intersperse among the type Ⅰ cells. They are also named secretary cells, having the ability of secretion of surfactant that plays an important role in reducing the surface tension at the air-epithelium interface and keeping the normal size of alveoli. Hyperplasia of type Ⅱ alveolar cells is an important marker of alveolar injury and repair of alveoli. After lung injury, they proliferate and restore both types of alveolar cells within the alveolus. (Fig. 5)

2) Alveolar septum: Alveoli are surrounded and separated from one another by an exceedingly thin connective tissue layer that contains collagen fibers, reticular fibers, elastic fibers, blood capillaries, fibroblasts and macrophages. The tissue between two airspaces is called alveolar septum. There are alveolar pores (10-15μm in diameter) in the interalveolar septa, allowing air to pass between alveoli. (Fig. 5)

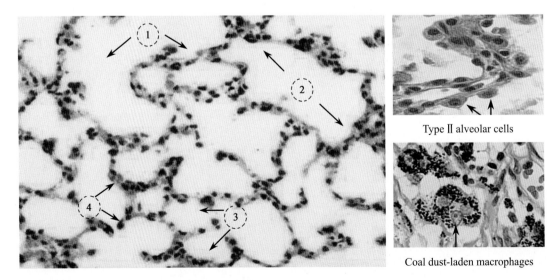

Type Ⅱ alveolar cells

Coal dust-laden macrophages

Fig. 5　Alveolar ducts (1), alveolar sacs (2), alveoli (3), alveolar septum (4)

3) Alveolar macrophages: Alveolar macrophages, located at the alveolar septum and airspace, are large (10-15μm in diameter), various-shaped cells with fingerlike projections on the surface. Macrophages display obvious evidence of phagocytotic activity, for example, visible ingested material (bacterium, foreign body, cell and its debris, dust, and so on) within their cytoplasm, playing an important protective role in removing small inhaled particles. After phagocytosis, the macrophages of alveolar space may be removed by the airway (mucus-cilia system), but hardly back to the alveolar septum since they become larger size and the decrease in migration; and the macrophages in alveolar septum can be removed by lymphatic draining or deposited in the interstitial tissue. (Fig. 5)

2.2   Mesenchyma: It contains blood vessels, lymphatic vessels and nerves.

2.2.1   Blood vessels: The lung has both pulmonary and bronchial circulations.

(1) Pulmonary circulations: It is the functional structure.

Characteristic: The pulmonary circulation is derived from the pulmonary artery that leaves the right ventricle of the heart, and supplies the capillaries of the alveolar septum which is the site of gas exchange. After gas exchange, blood is oxygenated and collected by pulmonary veins that return blood to the left atrium of the heart.

(2) Bronchial circulation: It is the nutritional structure.

The bronchial circulation, via bronchial arteries that branch from the aorta, supplies the capillaries of all the lung tissue (such as bronchi, bronchioles, alveoli, pulmonary lymph nodes, pleura, pulmonary blood vessels, and connective tissue).

The branches of the pulmonary artery travel with those of the bronchi and bronchioles and carry blood down to the capillary level at the alveoli. Therefore, anastomosis between bronchial and pulmonary circulations causes multiple derivations of blood of the pulmonary lobule with different types.

2.2.2   Pulmonary lymphatic vessels: They are divided into two groups.

(1) Superficial lymphatic vessels: This set of lymphatic vessels travels in the connective tissue of the visceral pleura, forming a dense network of lymphatic vessels that brings lymph into several larger lymphatic vessels and finally into hilar lymph nodes.

(2) Deep lymphatic vessels: Deep lymphatic vessels travel in the wall of bronchial tree, around pulmonary capillaries and in the connective tissue of interlobular septum. Juxtaalveolar lymphatic vessels locate at the alveolar septum which is adjacent to pleura, bronchi, blood vessels and interlobular septum. All of them drain lymph into several larger lymphatic vessels and finally into hilar lymph nodes. The lymph of hilum, via broncho-tracheal lymph nodes, paratracheal lymph node, enters the right lymphatic trunk; while the lymphatic vessels directly drain the upper lobe of the right lung or part of them, to the thoracic duct. There are anastomotic branches between the right lymphatic trunk and the thoracic duct, by which lymph moves from one part to another with high pressure.

(3) Histology of lymphatic vessels

1) Lymphatic capillaries: Lymphatic capillaries that are not visible at the level of the light microscope are lined with endothelial cells and have no cells in lumen. Since endothelial cells joint to others loosely and are lack of continuous basement membrane, the walls of the lymphatic capillaries are more permeable than the walls of blood capillaries; large molecules gain entry more readily into the lymphatic capillaries than into blood capillaries.

2) Collected lymphatic vessels: The collected lymphatic vessels are lined with regular endothelial cells with occluding junction, but are still lack of continuous basement membrane. The wall becomes a little thicker, due to the increase in connective tissue and bundles of smooth muscle. Lymphatic vessels possess valves that prevent backflow of lymph, thus aiding unidirectional flow.

2.2.3 Pulmonary nerves: Pulmonary plexus is composed of the sympathetic and vagal divisions of the autonomic nervous system. The innervation of branches of pulmonary plexus is consistent with bronchi.

1) Vagus nerve: They are the cholinergic nerve fibers, whose nerve endings located at smooth muscle cells, glands, and vessels of bronchial tree. They modify the dimensions of the air passages and blood flow by contraction of the smooth muscle in their walls, and promote the secretion of glands.

2) Sympathetic nerve: They are the adrenergic nerve fibers, whose nerve endings also located at smooth muscle cells, glands, and vessels of bronchial tree. They regulate the relaxation of smooth muscle in their walls, contraction of blood vessels, and inhibit the secretion of glands.

3) Sensory nerve fibers: They are located in the mucosa of bronchi, pulmonary connective tissue, visceral pleura, and around the alveolar epithelial cells, traveling within vagus nerve fibers. They are the sites of stretching perception.

(Ying Sun, Zhong-Qiu Wei)

Part II

Pathology of Coal Workers' Pneumoconiosis

Coal workers' pneumoconiosis (commonly referred to as coal mines' pneumoconiosis) is a chronic occupational pulmonary disease caused by long-term inhalation of coal mine dust. Variation of occupational environment, such as geographical conditions of coal mine industries, work types of coal miners, respiratory coal mine dusts (coal dusts, silica, or combination of coal dusts and silica), pulmonary infective diseases, cause a spectrum of pulmonary morphological changes, now known to include anthracosilicosis, silicosis and anthracosis.

In coal mine industry, the coal miners who perform rock drilling or rock transportion may be induced to silicosis, due to exposure of high concentration of respirable crystalline free silica (it is about 30% of respirable coal mine dust); if these coal miners continue to expose respirable coal mine dust deposited in lung, their silicosis are referred to combination of silicosis and anthracosis, which histologic changes are similar as silicosis. Coal mine dust that are usually exposed to underground hewer, transport workers, timberer, stevedore (works in surface coal bunker), coal-washing worker, contains more coal dust and less crystalline free silica (< 10% of respirable coal mine dust), who may have anthracosis if they keep their work type. In fact, the simple anthracosis is rare since the coal miners usually change their job and expose to both coal dust and silica. In China, the common type of coal works' pneumoconiosis is anthracosilicosis, which is consistent with our findings based on the 47 cases of autopsy specimens; and both the simple silicosis and the simple anthracosis are rare.

1 Gross appearance of coal workers' pneumoconiosis [1,3,12]

1.1 Coal dust maculae: It contains pleural coal dust maculae and pulmonary coal dust maculae.

Coal dust maculae is the most common type of coal workers' pneumoconiosis, defined as a collection of coal dust particles in the vesicle pleura and in pulmonary tissue, with diameter arranged from 3mm to 5mm. In the microscopic view or large slice of whole lung, maculae can be divided into coal dust dots and coal dust foci dependent on the formation of consolidated lesions. However, this difference is hardly to be found at the level of gross appearance.

1.1.1　Pleural coal dust maculae: Various-sized, round or quasi-circular, black maculae which diameters arrange from 3mm to 5mm are widely distributed on the visceral pleural surface. The soft maculae are well demarcated from the surrounding tissue, representing the border of pulmonary lobules due to coal dust deposits at the interface between pleura and interlobular septum.

1.1.2　Pulmonary coal dust maculae: On the cut surface of lungs, the black maculae are similar as pleural maculae, but usually surrounded by a halo of centriacinar (focal) emphysema in a black cystic fashion (3mm-5mm in diameter), looking like sponge. Maculae are sharply delimited from the surrounding tissue when they distribute loosely; otherwise the border become unclear.

In the large slice of whole lung, coal dust foci are differentiated from coal dust dots by a preponderance of consolidated lesions. Sometimes, a coal dust nodule, showing a round or stary, more than 5mm in diameter, black, hard (like rubber) appearance, could be seen in the case of a large amount of coal dust foci in lung.

1.2　Coal dust nodules: It contains coal (silicotic) nodules and silicotic (coal) nodules.

In our specimens, all nodular lesions display the round or quasi-circular, black appearance, ranging the diameter from 2mm to 5mm. This gross appearance is no benefit to distinguish coal (silicotic) nodules from silicotic (coal) nodules.

1.2.1　Coal (silicotic) nodules (coal silicotic nodules): They show round or oval, gray-black, hard appearance with 3 mm-5mm in diameter, and are differentiated from silicotic (coal) nodules by a central core of collagen, with a peripheral stellate component of greater coal dust deposits.

1.2.2　Silicotic (coal) nodules (silicotic nodules): The classic silicotic (coal) nodules, usually showing a round or oval, gray-black, hard appearance with 2 mm-3mm in diameter, are rarely present in the lung with coal workers' pneumoconiosis.

1.3　Massive fibrosis: It contains progressive massive fibrosis, nodular confluent massive fibrosis, and combination of progressive massive fibrosis and nodular confluent massive fibrosis.

1.3.1　Progressive massive fibrosis: It shows a large (greater than 2cm*2cm*2cm in volume), firm, black lesion, with destruction of bronchi and blood vessels or slit-shaped cavities created by tissue necrosis.

1.3.2　Nodular confluent massive fibrosis: It shows a large (greater than 2cm*2cm*2cm in volume), stony-hard, black lesion, with the coalescence response of round or quasi-circular nodules.

1.3.3   Combination of progressive massive fibrosis and nodular confluent massive fibrosis: The lung shows a large (greater than 2cm*2cm*2cm in volume), firm, black lesion where progressive massive fibrosis is admixed with nodular confluent massive fibrosis.

Comment: Massive fibrosis was previously classified, according to the development of lesion, with progressive massive fibrosis and nodular confluent massive fibrosis. However, our samples do reveal the concurrence of nodular fusion and progressive massive fibrosis. So, here we point out the new type of massive fibrosis—combination of progressive massive fibrosis and nodular confluent massive fibrosis.

1.4   Diffuse interstitial fibrosis

The changes of diffuse interstitial fibrosis are common in coal workers' pneumoconiosis, showing characteristic drooping willows and cords of fibrous tissue, loss of normal tissue.

1.5   Emphysema

Emphysema is predominantly around the black coal dust maculae and coal silicotic nodules, showing various-sized cysts. Sometimes, the cystlike structure is advanced to bullae (more than 1cm in diameter) with the residual blood vessels or fibrous tissue hanging on the wall, as the consequence of destruction of alveolar septa.

1.6   Lesions in the lymph nodes (usually in hilar lymph nodes)

The involved lymph node becomes larger, firm and black, with a patchy area of chalky white responded to calcification. Sometimes, the lymph node may be essentially converted to eggshell-like stone in the cases of severe calcification.

1.7   Lesions in pleura

Adhesion and thickening are the common process when pleura are involved. In time, hyaline change or bone metaplasia appears in the focus of adhesion and thickening, showing a stony-hard, glassy, pale appearance (like cartilage tissue).

1.8   Coal works' pneumoconiosis with tuberculosis

1.8.1   Coal dust maculae with disseminated miliary tuberculosis: Scattered black coal dust maculae are mixed with military pale caseous necrosis in whole lung.

1.8.2   Massive fibrosis with disseminated miliary tuberculosis: The upper lobe of the left lung reveals a diffusely consolidated, pale, cheesy appearance, in which the black fibrous lesions studded with pale caseous necrosis are adjacent to the interlobar fissure. The lower lobe of the left lung is riddle with pale areas of disseminated miliary tuberculosis (illustrated by Fig.31 and Fig.32).

1.8.3 Coal works' pneumoconiosis with tuberculosis in hilar lymph nodes: The enlarged hilar lymph nodes have coal dust deposition and caseous necrosis.

1.9 Coal works' pneumoconiosis with lung cancer

1.9.1 Coal works' pneumoconiosis with lung cancer (Peripheral type): A round or quasi-circular, gray-yellow, cheesy tumor mass is visible in lung with coal works' pneumoconiosis.

1.9.2 Coal works' pneumoconiosis with lung cancer (Diffuse type): Coal dust-deposited lung provides the evidence of multiple widespread tumor masses, characterized by gray-yellow color and different size.

1.10 Coal works' pneumoconiosis with cor pulmonale

Cor pulmonale consists of right ventricular hypertrophy and dilation due to pulmonary hypertension caused by disorders of the lung parachyma or pulmonary vasculature which are usually induced by chronic diseases.

The heart has an increase in mass and weight, associated with blunt apex and bulged pulmonary conus arteriosus. The right ventricle reveals characteristics of hypertrophy and dilation, showing thickened wall and hypertrophied partial trabeculae carneae and papillary muscle.

(Hong Xu, He-Liang Liu)

2 Histological changes of coal workers' pneumoconiosis [1-12]

2.1 Anthracosilicosis

2.1.1 Coal dust dots: According to the anatomic distribution, coal dust dots are classified into pleural coal dust dots and pulmonary coal dust dots.

(1) Pleural coal dust dots: The black maculae, predominantly localized to pleura, subpleura, interface between pleura and interlobular septum, are packed with coal dust-laden macrophages, surrounded by minimal reticular fibers or collagen fibers.

(2) Pulmonary coal dust dots: It is a special type of coal workers' pneumoconiosis, being a collective process of coal dust-laden macrophages along the small bronchia, bronchioles, respiratory bronchioles and their airspaces, small blood vessels. Note no consolidated lesions, but most often association with centriacinar emphysema.

2.1.2 Coal dust foci: Coal dust foci are created by long-time accumulation of coal dust-laden macrophages around small bronchia, bronchioles, respiratory bronchioles, and small blood vessels. Moreover, macrophages with coal dust have so strong ability in movement that they could arrive at the terminal blind alveoli. However, excessive deposits of coal dust can cause emphysema due to obstruction of small airway.

Characeristic histological appearance of coal dust foci is consolidated center of coal dust-laden macrophages and/or proliferated fibrous tissue surrounded by emphysema, which is the main difference from coal dust dots. Coal dust foci are also highlighted with various-shaped center (starry, crab-like, starfish-like, fish-like, horse-like, bird-like, and so on). According to the content of fibrous tissue, coal dust foci could be classified into two types: cellular coal dust foci and fibrous coal dust foci.

(1) Cellular coal dust foci: The various-shaped black foci are composed of abundant coal dust-laden macrophages, less collagen fibers, and minimal reticular fibers (be visible with silver stain), accompanied with obstructive emphysema.

(2) Fibrous coal dust foci: Compared with cellular coal dust foci, the lesions of fibrous coal dust foci have much more amount of collagen fibers (less than 50% of the lesion) in a cord pattern.

2.1.3   Nodular lesion: According to the development, it could be classified with cellular nodules, cellular fibrous nodules, and fibrous nodules.

(1) Macrophage alveolitis: Inhalation of the exogenous stimuli (dust, chemical agents, physical agents, infectious agents) could trigger macrophage predominant inflammation of the alveoli.

The onset is abundant neutrophils with proteinaceous fluid, infiltrated in the alveolar spaces. With the replacement of neutrophils by macrophages, the alveolar spaces are packed with much more macrophages, occasional neutrophils, detached epithelial cells and others, forming macrophage alveolitis. Phagocytosis of the inhaled coal dust facilitates coal dust depositing in macrophage cytoplasm, macrophage being larger. Furthermore, a collection of coal dust-laden macrophages in the alveoli is regarded as the basis of nodular granuloma, which could finally develop to cellular coal dust nodules.

(2) Cellular coal dust nodules: Cells with coal dust aggregate in the alveolar spaces, forming multiple round or quasi-circular nodules (Granuloma in response to coal dust). Minimal collagen fibers between cells are visible.

(3) Cellular fibrous coal dust nodules: In this stage, fibroblasts between coal dust-laden macrophages start to proliferate and produce modest collagen fibers.

(4) Fibrous coal dust nodules: Besides of a large amount of coal dust-laden macrophages, the nodules contain abundant collagen fibers in a cord or bundle pattern. The center of nodule is characterized by the hyaline collagenous tissue arranged in a laminated pattern, coal dust deposits heavily enclosing the lesion, forming a "cuff-cover" appearance. The fibrous tissue protrudes from the lesion and extends into surrounding tissue, creating many hair-shaped pseudopodia. This fibrous coal dust nodule is referred as typical coal silicotic nodule.

Comment: ①In contrast to silicotic coal nodule, coal silicotic nodule reveals a small core composed by less collagen fibers and coal dust, more coal dust deposits in the periphery (the area that coal dust occupied is over one third of whole lesion), and many hair shaped pseudopodia spreading to the surrounding tissue. ②In coal workers' pneumoconiosis, between clearly fibrous coal dust foci and obvious nodular lesions are borderline fibrous coal dust foci (atypical coal silicotic nodules), showing a consolidated, various-shaped (starry, polygonal, irregular), mildly larger (more than 5mm in diameter) lesion. Histologically, storiform pattern of proliferated fibrous tissue is over 50% of whole lesion, with scattered distribution of coal dust-laden macrophages. The pseudopodia-shaped fibrous tissue frequently protrudes from the lesion, spreading along the interstitial tissue.

2.1.4　Massive fibrosis: Massive fibrosis is common in anthracosilicosis with stage Ⅲ, characterized by a large size (greater than 2cm*2cm*2cm in volume), containing abundant coal dust deposits, pulmonary debris, and necrotic coal dust cavity. It is classified into progressive massive fibrosis, confluent nodular massive fibrosis, combination of progressive massive fibrosis and confluent nodular massive fibrosis.

(1) Progressive massive fibrosis: Diffuse fibrous proliferation and deposits of coal dust form an extensive mass, frequently including "coal dust pool" which is the mixture of abundant coal dust deposits and necrotic debris.

(2) Confluent nodular massive fibrosis: The massive lesion is created by coalescence of multiple coal silicotic nodules with scattered distribution of coal dust-laden macrophages.

(3) Combination of progressive massive fibrosis and confluent nodular massive fibrosis: it is a process that progressive massive fibrosis undergoes the coalescence response with confluent nodular massive fibrosis.

2.1.5　Coal interstitial fibrosis: After coal dust and coal dust-laden macrophages deposition along pleura, interlobular septum, airway, small bronchia, bronchioles, and small blood vessels, the pulmonary tissue are destroyed, in turn interstitial fibroblasts start to proliferate and produce excessive collagen, finally forming a diffuse fibrous net in lung. Indeed, coal interstitial fibrosis is more often in anthracosilicosis, that is why "once coal dust deposition, always interstitial fibrosis formation". Sometimes, interstitial smooth muscle cells get to proliferation too.

Onset of coal interstitial fibrosis is in the respiratory bronchioles, then it spreads widely along alveolar septum, interlobular septum, small bronchia, bronchioles, and small blood vessels, forming a crablike feet appearance. The interlobular septum becomes thickening when the proliferative response occurs in the interlobular septum, do the same as pleura. A large amount of coal dust deposits make coal interstitial fibrosis to be black color, which is the main difference from metallic dust pneumoconiosis.

(Fang Yang, Ying Sun)

2.2　Silicosis

2.2.1　Macrophage alveolitis: The basic changes of macrophage alveolitis in silicosis are same as the one in anthracosilicosis, except that silica-laden macrophage is not black color.

2.2.2　Silicotic (coal) nodules (silicotic nodules): The nodules are as large as 0.2mm to 1.5mm in diameter. H.E section of the typical nodules is central proliferated collagen fibers in a laminated pattern with hyaline change, showing homogenous red color. Masson stain highlights the collagen as blue color, which indeed includes collagen type Ⅰ stained by Sirius red stain with orange color and collagen type III showed green color (polarized light microscope). In addition, a variable amount of coal dust deposits locates to the periphery of nodules or around the lesions.

It is worth mentioning that the typical silicotic (coal) nodules are hardly seen in coal workers' pneumoconiosis. The characteristic of coal silicotic nodules that is different from silicotic (coal) nodules is the obvious deposition of coal dust, surrounding the center of nodules. However, single morphological difference has no benefit on distinguishing coal silicotic nodules and silicotic (coal) nodules. Here, we define as coal silicotic nodules if the area of coal dust deposits (usually being the "cuff-cover" structure) is more than 1/3 of the lesion or there are pseudopodia-shaped fibrous tissue, while silicotic (coal) nodules when less coal dust deposits (the area of coal dust deposits is less than 1/3 of the lesion, or not circumferential).

Silicotic nodules are more common in the lymph nodes, probably due to the more consolidated consistency compared with lung tissue.

2.2.3　Massive fibrosis: Massive fibrosis is a coalescent process of silicotic nodules, characterized by a clear border zoom of each small silicotic nodule with hyaline change, frequently with collapsed or destructed small bronchi, bronchioles, small blood vessels and alveoli. Between the confluent massive fibrous lesions is the proliferated fibrous tissue with coal dust deposition.

Comments: Massive fibrosis of silicosis is mainly created by fusion of silicotic nodules, associated with variable amount of fibrous tissue. Progressive massive fibrosis is rare in silicosis, which is the difference from anthracosilicosis.

2.2.4　Dust interstitial fibrosis: The basic changes of interstitial fibrosis induced by silica are similar as the one induced by coal dust, but the response is much more severe, probably due to the hardness of silica particles.

2.3　Anthracosis

It is still arguing that coal dust without silica particles could induce coal workers' pneumoconiosis. So, it should be careful to diagnose with anthracosis in clinic.

However, coal dust, mixed with a few amounts of silica particles, do cause coal workers' pneumoconiosis in both lung and lymph nodes, evidenced by coal dust dots, coal dust foci, emphysema around the coal dust foci, coal interstitial fibrosis, and so on; note: no formation of type nodular lesions (sillicotic nodules and coal silicotic nodules).

Histologically, coal dust dots, coal dust foci, centriacinar emphysema are visible in lung, with variable amount of proliferated interstitial fibrous tissue. Gross view of pleura and lung shows abundant black maculae or confluent maculae, usually surrounded by centriacinar emphysema. Sometimes, coal dust deposits so seriously that the whole lung becomes uniformly black. The involved lymph nodes are enlarging, tender, black, with presentation of a large amount of coal dust deposits and mild interstitial fibrosis microscopically.

(He-Liang Liu, Hong Xu)

2.4 Complicated lesions

2.4.1 Pulmonary tuberculosis[21-24]: It keeps consistency between coal works' pneumoconiosis and pulmonary tuberculosis, evidenced by 75% of tuberculosis incidence in the patients of coal works' pneumoconiosis with stage III. Tuberculosis further aggravates coal works' pneumoconiosis. In the cases of coal works' pneumoconiosis with tuberculosis, invasion into a bronchus evacuates the caseous necrosis, creating a tuberculosis cavity, and aggressiveness of blood vessels induces severe bleeding, causing people death. According to the histological features, there are two types of tuberculosis in coal works' pneumoconiosis: separated type and confluent type.

(1) Separated type: The distinctive feature of this type tuberculosis is well preservation of morphological changes of tuberculosis and the co-existed coal works' pneumoconiosis; for example, the lung could reveal characteristic coal silicotic nodules and tubercles in the case of coal works' pneumoconiosis with tuberculosis (Separated type).

(2) Confluent type: In this type of tuberculosis, tuberculosis lesion merges with coal works' pneumoconiosis, with loss of its individual morphological changes, but forming a larger lesions (coal silicotic tuberculous nodule).

The larger-sized coal silicotic tuberculous nodule is enclosed by a large amount of fibrous tissue, coal dust deposition within or surrounded the nodule; and the center of nodule is extensive caseous necrosis, often with coal silicotic nodules debris, scattered coal dust-laden macrophages, and free coal dust deposits. In general, caseous necrosis is commonly seen in coal silicotic tuberculous nodule, but epithelioid cells, Langhans' giant cells and lymphocytes are seldom involved. However, sometimes caseous necrosis with fewer epithelioid cells, atypical giant cells and lymphocytes could be seen.

In favorable cases, a focus with exudation and/or tubercles, surrounded the coal silicotic tuberculous nodule, undergoes the changes of coalescence, necrosis, fibrous encapsulation, forming a larger coal silicotic tuberculous nodule. The coalescence actions of coal silicotic tuberculous nodules, tubercles, coal silicotic nodules, and other coal lesions could facilitate the progressiveness of coal works' pneumoconiosis, and during which tuberculosis cavity is easily created.

Coal bronchitis may advance coal tuberculous bronchitis, when tuberculosis affects bronchus, showing caseation in the background of coal bronchitis.

It is worth mentioning that pulmonary tuberculosis makes coal works' pneumoconiosis to be more complex. The lung displays the marked pleomorphism, and there are other changes that not shown here.

2.4.2 Lung tumor[25-29]: Coal works' pneumoconiosis facilities the carcinogenesis, due to the similar roles of coal dusts as carcinogenic agents. Therefore, lung cancer, such as small-cell carcinoma, adenocarcinoma, squamous cell carcinoma, adenosquamous carcinoma, and other malignant cancers (such as malignant mesothelioma) may be present in the cases of coal works' pneumoconiosis.

2.5   Others

Coal dust in lung could be removed via lymphatic system. howevert, when coal dust reaches at lymph nodes with lymph flow, it could destruct lymph nodes and stimulates fibrous proliferation; furthermore it may invade the surrounded tissue (organ) via penetration into the capsule of lymph nodes, inducing loss of normal structure and dysfunction. Here we will list the commonly involved sites or changes, base on our specimens.

2.5.1   Lesions of lymph nodes: Coal dust in lung travels along the superficial lymphatic vessels or deep lymphatic vessels, finally reaching at pleural lymph nodes and perivascular lymph nodes, especially at hilar lymph nodes, subfornix lymph nodes, and parabronchial lymph nodes. There, the lesions induced by coal dust are classified into coal dust deposition, fibrous proliferation and fibrosis as well as nodular foci.

(1) Coal dust deposition: Coal dust-laden macrophages firstly deposit in medulla where cause tissue necrosis, and continue extending to the cortex. Between the cells with coal dust are the proliferated reticular fibers.

(2) Fibrous proliferation: The deposited coal dust stimulates fibroblasts and fibrous tissue proliferation, creating a focus of fibrous tissue with loss of normal structure.

(3) Nodular foci: Nodular foci are based on coal dust deposition and coal fibrosis, including cellular nodules, cellular fibrous nodules and fibrous nodules.

(4) Lymph nodes (such as hilar lymph nodes, parabronchial lymph nodes) are the favorite sites of coal work's pneumoconiosis with tuberculosis, in which the changes induced by coal dust (such as coal silicotic nodules, interstitial fibrosis) and the lesions of tuberculosis co-exist, and/or merge into a larger focus (coal silicotic tuberculous nodule). Sometimes, the coalescence action of coal silicotic tuberculous nodules is so severe that it could create a big nodule with wide destruction of normal structure.

2.5.2   Lesions of bronchi: Coal work's pneumoconiosis could influence main bronchi or lobar bronchi, evidenced by the replacement of bronchial wall by coal fibrous tissue containing fibroblasts (including myofibroblasts), moderate amount of collagen fibers, and scattered coal dust-laden macrophages. The infiltrating mode of coal fibrous tissue facilitate it to invade bronchi from adventitia to mucosa, showing a polypoid penetrating into mucosa, a separation of glands or ducts in submucosa with gland atrophy, a loss of cartilage tissue via penetration of cartilage capsule, or a localized nodule in the bronchial wall.

Coal work's pneumoconiosis is more often accompanied by bronchitis, which is named with coal bronchitis. Characteristic histological features of coal bronchitis contain mucus hyperplasia, hypertrophy and hypersecretion, goblet cells proliferation, mucus plugging of bronchiolar lumen, occasional replacement of mucosal epithelial cells by squamous metaplasia, inflammation with a variable density of lymphocytes in submucosa with scattered coal dust-laden macrophages. In the severe cases, coal fibrous tissue penetrates into the bronchial wall, producing bronchial debris. In addition, although coal dust-laden macrophages accumulate in the adventitia of both large airway and small airway, respiratory bronchioles is the most favorite sites.

It should be emphasized that chronic bronchitis with fibrous proliferation in bronchial wall is often prior to coal bronchitis. So it is difficult to distingue who mainly contributes to the fibrosis response, coal dust deposits or chronic inflammation.

2.5.3　Lesions of pleura: Coal dust close to the pleura, via lymph flow, is delivered to pleura, where the deposited coal dust not only extends along the interlobular septum, revealing the outline of pulmonary lobules clearly and forming pleural and subpleural coal maculae, but also stimulates subpleural small blood vessels congestion and hyperplasia as well as fibrous proliferation, leading to pleural thickening and adhesion. Sometimes, occasional coal silicotic nodules or tissue debris are visible in the thicken pleura.

2.5.4　Emphysema in response to coal dust: Coal dust deposited in bronchi stimulates the bronchial wall thickening, even and narrowing of the lumen. While coal dust deposited in terminal bronchiole and its distal parts (respiratory bronchioles, alveolar ducts, alveolar sacs, alveoli) creates large airspace and destructs the alveolar septum, leading to emphysema. Centriacinar emphysema is common in coal work's pneumoconiosis, characterized by the located at central lobule large airspace, surrounding coal dust maculae or coal dust foci. In severe cases, respiratory bronchioles, alveolar ducts and alveolar sacs are uniformly enlarged, and destructive panacinar emphysema is visible, showing a black cyst with 1cm in diameter, remained small blood vessel and bridge-shaped fibrous tissue hanging on the wall. It could further advance to bullae.

2.5.5　Lesions of small blood vessels: Coal dust deposits in arteries and veins of the lung. In arteries, coal fibrous tissue invades from adeventitia to medium, destroying the normal structure (elastic fibers rupture). Since the venous wall is thin, coal fibrous tissue is ability to penetrate all layers, causing an uneven intima and a black wall. Sometimes, these small vessels with thrombus in lumen could be entrapped to coal nodular lesions, and coal dust that invades into the lumen may admix with blood cells.

2.5.6　Lesions of adipose tissue: Coal dust extends to the adjacent adipose tissue from the bronchial adventitia, evidenced by abundant coal dust-laden macrophages deposition in adipose tissue, accompanied with interstitial fibrous proliferation and small blood vessels proliferation and congestion.

2.5.7　Lesions of lymphatic vessels: Lymph flow plays a very important role in removing the inhaled coal dust. Coal dust cause lymphatic vessels dilation, deposits in lumen and thickens the vessels wall.

2.5.8　Lesions of nerves: Coal dust deposited in lung or bronchi may invade nerve trunk by penetration into the surrounding membrane.

2.5.9　Pulmonary infection: Coal dust causes defect in innate immunity, which increases incidence of infection of bacteria, virus and others, inducing pulmonary infection (such as suppurative inflammation, serous inflammation, fibrinous inflammation, mixed inflammation).

2.5.10   "Rod-shaped" body [9]: "Rod-shaped" body is common in our samples. The rod-shaped, dumbbell-shaped, fascicular or bead-shaped bodies are 15 to 50μm in length, the center with black color or strong power of refraction. Freedom or cluster of "rod-shaped" bodies is widely distributed in alveolar space, alveolar septum, coal dust foci, coal silicotic nodules, and fibrous interstitial tissue. However, the pathogenesis keeps unclear. Li HZ had documented that the formation of "rod-shaped" body is similar as the one of asbestos body of asbestosis. It is rich in ferritin, naming as "ferruginous body". It is possibly related to macrophages accumulation, type II alveolar cells proliferation, and interstitial fibrosis.

2.5.11   Myofibroblast differentiation [33-37]: Years of stimui that promote fibrous proliferation causes transformation of mucosal epithelial cells and interstitial fibroblasts into myofibroblasts with α-smooth muscle actin (α-SMA) expression, as a key step to facilitate the formation of pulmonary fibrosis. We have documented that myofibroblasts do be present in the nodular lesions and interstitial fibrous tissue of coal work's pneumoconiosis, and evidence of origin discovers the interstitial fibroblasts and type II alveolar cells using animal model of silicosis.

2.5.12   Cor pulmonale: Twenty one cases of forty seven autopsy samples record the changes of lung and heart, of which there are nine cases with right ventricular hypertrophy and dilation. Microscopically, myocyte of right ventricular has an increased diameter, associated with prominent irregular nuclear enlargement. The patchy areas of necrotic tissue could be seen in the right ventricle, some of which are replaced by dense collagenous scar, with edema and fibrous proliferation in the interstitial tissue.

In addition, coal dusts could reach at and deposit in the other organs (such as spleen, liver) via blood flow.

(Xu-Dong Song, Zhong-Qiu Wei, Fang Yang)

References

[1] Li HZ, Li TS. Relationship between pathological changes and pathological diagnosis of anthracosilicosis based on 120 coal miners [J]. Zhi Ye Wei Sheng Yu Bing Shang, 1989, 4 (1): 1-4.

[2] Li TS, Li HZ. Pathological observation of interstitial sclerosis slicosis [J]. Zhong Guo Zong He Lin Chuang, 1980, 1: 30-35.

[3] Li HZ, Li TS. Pathological types of coal works' pneumoconiosis [J]. Mei Kuang Yi Xue, 1982, 4 (Suppl): 72-74.

[4] Li HZ, Li TS. Pathological morphology criteria of coal works' pneumoconiosis [J]. Mei Kuang Yi Xue, 1982, 4 (Suppl): 69-71.

[5] Li HZ, Li TS. Basic pathological changes of coal works' pneumoconiosis [J]. Mei Kuang Yi Xue, 1982, 4 (Suppl): 65-68.

[6] Li TS, Li HZ. Nodular lesions observation of coal works' pneumoconiosis [J]. Mei Kuang Yi Xue, 1981, 3 (2): 1-4.

[7] Li HZ, Li TS. Productive coal dust deposition in lungs [J]. Mei Kuang Yi Xue, 1981, 3 (3): 31-35.

[8] Li TS, Li HZ. Effect of pulmonary complications on coal works' pneumoconiosis [J]. Mei Kuang Yi Xue,

1982,4(Suppl):75-77.

[9] Li HZ,Wang HY,Meng SG,et al. Morphology observation of ferruginous body and the characteristics of coal works' pneumoconiosis [J]. Zhong Hua Bing Li Za Zhi,1991,20(3):169-171.

[10] Li HZ,Li TS. Pulmonary Morphological changes induced by the mixture of coal dust and silica in rats [J]. Zhi Ye Wei Sheng Yu Bing Shang,1989,4(3):7-12.

[11] Wang XH,Li TS,Yang F,et al. The therapy effect of Yantai on the experimental anthracosis in rats with long-time exposure to coal dust [J]. Zhong Guo Mei Tan Gong Ye Yi Xue Za Zhi,1998,5(1):477-479.

[12] Li HZ,Li TS. Histological atlas of coal works' pneumoconiosis [M]. Beijing:Energy Press,1987.

[13] Dai YF,Qin LG,Zhang ZW. Analysis of projects funded by the National Natural Science Foundation of China in the field of occupational health and occupational diseases from 2010 to 2017 [J]. Zhong Hua Yu Fang Yi Xue Za Zhi,2018,52(7):769-771.

[14] Han B,Liu HB,Zhai GJ,et al. Estimates and predictions of coal workers' pneumoconiosis cases among redeployed coal workers of the Fuxin Mining Industry Group in China:A historical cohort study [J]. PLos One,2016,11(2):e0148179.

[15] Cheng BW,Su M. International incidence trend of coal workers' pneumoconiosis [J]. Zhong Hua Lao Dong Wei Sheng Zhi Ye Bing Za Zhi,2019,37(1):75-78.

[16] Han S,Chen H,Harvey MA,et al. Focusing on coal workers' lung diseases:a comparative analysis of China,Australia,and the United States [J]. Int J Environ Res Public Health,2018,15(11).:E2565.

[17] China Coal Industry Association. Annual report on coal industry development in 2017. March 27,2018.

[18] National Statistical Office. Third national economic census. March 1,2016.

[19] Li DH. Do not misleading the prevention and treatment of pneumoconiosis [J]. Huan Jing Yu Zhi Ye Wei Sheng,2018,35(4):283-285.

[20] Health Commission of the People's Republic of China. http://www.nhc.gov.cn/guihuaxxs/s10748/201905/9b8d52727cf346049de8acce25ffcbd0.shtml.

[21] Meng SG. Prevention and treatment of silicosis and tuberculosis in coal mine industries [M]. Beijing:Energy Press,1985.

[22] Yang F. Pathology of pulmonary tuberculosis in the cases of coal work's pneumoconiosis [M]//Ming Zhong.Pneumoconiosis complications. Bei Jing:China Medical Science Press,1993:45-48.

[23] Yew WW,Leung CC,Chang KC,et al. Can treatment outcomes of latent TB infection and TB in silicosis be improved?[J].J Thorac Dis,2019,11(1):E8-E10.

[24] Skowroński M1,Halicka A,Barinow-Wojewódzki A. Pulmonary tuberculosis in a male with silicosis [J]. Adv Respir Med,2018,86(3).

[25] Wang GH. Diagnosis and treatment of 31 cases of coal worker's pneumoconiosis with lung cancer [J]. Shi Yong Yi Yong Za Zhi,2010,17(3):258-259.

[26] Bao SW. Analysis of 38 cases of coal worker's pneumoconiosis with lung cancer [J]. Ji Lin Yi Xue,2012,33(18):3972.

[27] Manno M,Levy L,Johanson G,et al. Silicosis and lung cancer:what level of exposure is acceptable?[J]. Med Lav,2018,109(6):478-480.

[28] Sato T,Shimosato T,Klinman DM. Silicosis and lung cancer:current perspectives [J]. Lung Cancer,2018,9:91-101.

[29] Mlika M,Adigun R. Silicosis(Coal Worker Pneumoconiosis). Source stat pearls [Internet]. Treasure Island(FL):StatPearls Publishing. Jan 30,2019.

[30] Zhao PZ,Yang F. Pathobiological atlas of atherosclerosis in young Chinese [M]. Beijing:Concord Medical University Press,2006.

[31] Xu H, Yang F, Yuan Y, et al. Parameter selection for semi-quantitative analysis of immunohistochemical Image Pro Plus images [J]. Jie Pou Xue Za Zhi, 2012, 35 (1): 37-41.

[32] Yang F, Zhao PZ, She MP, et al. The relationship between the dynamic changes of several extracellular matrices and the formation of atherosclerosis in human coronary arteries [J]. Zhong Hua Bing Li Xue Za Zhi, 1998, 27 (3): 177-181.

[33] Zhang BN, Xu H, Zhang Y, et al. Targeting the RAS axis alleviates silicotic fibrosis and Ang II -inducedmyofibroblast differentiation via inhibition of the hedgehog signalingpathway [J]. Toxicology Letters, 2019, 313: 30-41.

[34] Zhang H, Xu DJ, Mao N, et al. Localization and expression of acetylated tubulin in silicotic fibroblasts [J]. Zhong Guo Zhi Ye Yi Xue, 2018, 45 (2): 150-156.

[35] Deng H, Xu H, Zhang X, et al. Protective effect of Ac-SDKP on alveolar epithelial cells through inhibition of EMT via TGF-β1/ROCK1 pathway in silicosis in rat [J]. Toxicol Appl Pharmacol, 2016, 16 (294): 1-10.

[36] Li SF, Xu H, Yi X, et al. Ac-SDKP increases α -TAT 1 and promotes the apoptosis in lung fibroblasts and epithelial cells double-stimulated with TGF-β1 and silica [J]. Toxicology and Applied Pharmacology, 2019, 369: 17-29.

[37] Su M, Zou CQ. Pathological diagnosis atlas of pneumoconiosis [M]. Bei Jing: People's Medical Publishing House, 2019.

[38] Zou ZZ, Li JC. Histology and Embryology [M].8th ed. Bei Jing: People's Medical Publishing House, 2013.

[39] Bo SL, Ying DJ. System of Anatomy [M].8th ed. Bei Jing: People's Medical Publishing House, 2013.

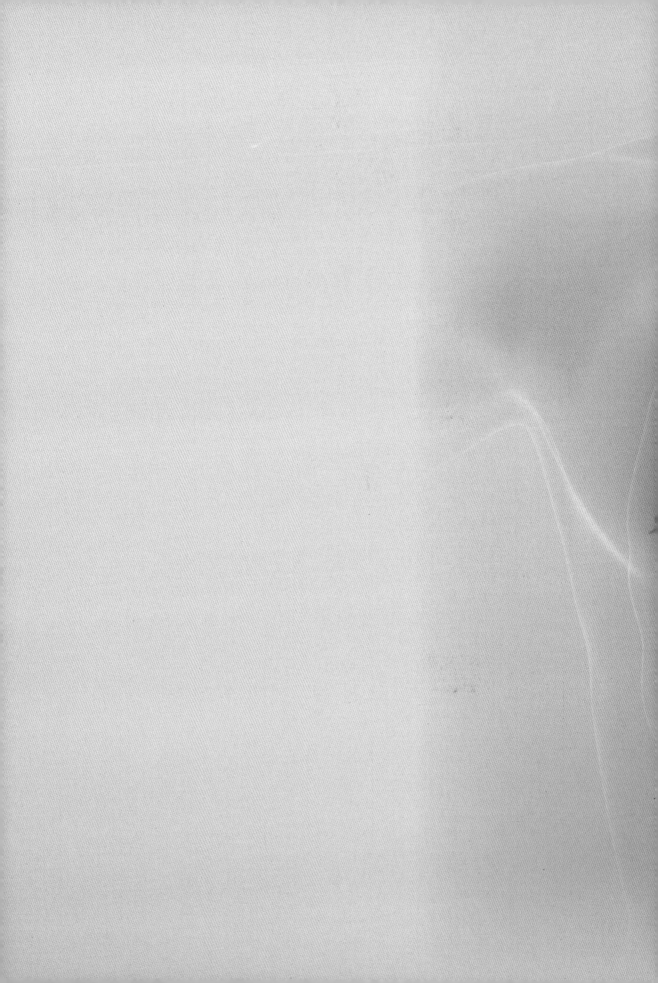

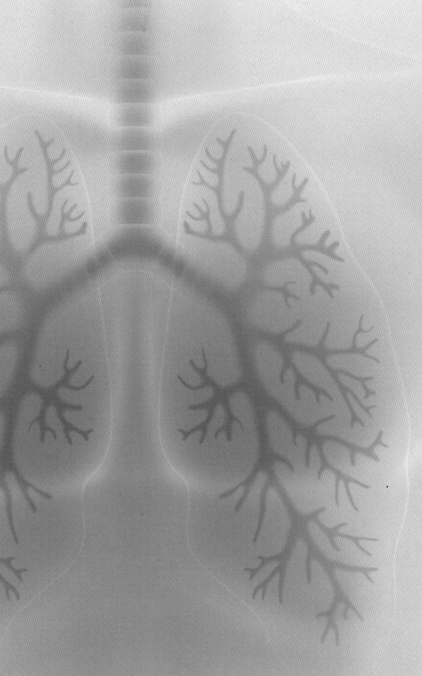

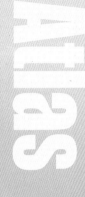

图谱部分

Atlas

第一部分
煤工尘肺大体形态学特点

Part I

Gross Appearance of Coal Workers' Pneumoconiosis

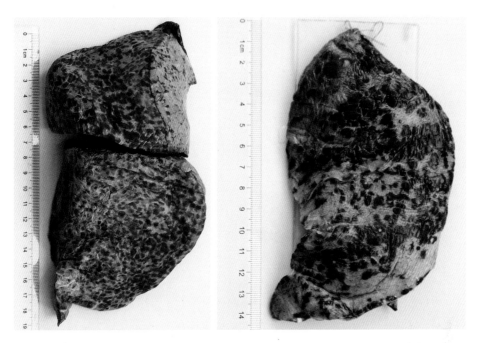

图 1 胸膜煤斑灶：肺表面可见圆形或类圆形黑色斑灶样病变，3~5mm，边界清晰，局部可融合成片。（掘进工作和其他井下工作 38 年）

Fig.1 Pleural coal dust maculae: Numerous round or quasi-circular black maculae 3-5 mm in diameter are widely distributed on the pleural surface. The maculae are well demarcated, but some of them get coalescence. (From the patient, performing coal tunneling and other underground work for 38 years)

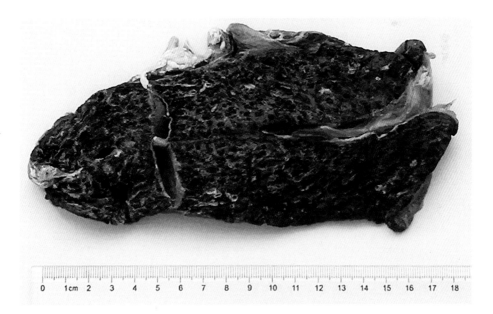

图 2 肺内煤斑灶：肺切面可见黑色斑灶样病变。（掘进、采煤工作 23 年）

Fig.2 Pulmonary coal dust maculae: Numerous round or quasi-circular black maculae on the cut surface of lung. (From the patient, working in coal tunneling and mining for 23 years)

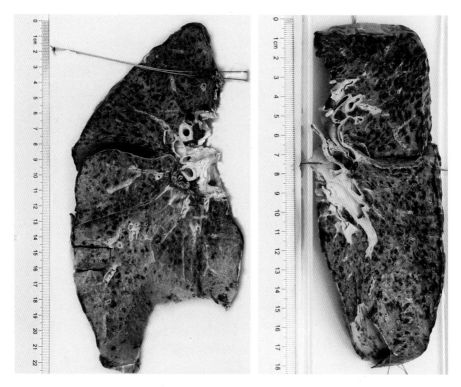

图 3　肺内煤斑灶：肺切面可见较多黑色斑灶样病变。肺门淋巴结肿大伴煤尘沉积。(井下运输工作 25 年)

Fig.3　Pulmonary coal dust maculae: The cut surface of lung shows lots of black maculae. Enlarged hilar lymph nodes with coal dust deposits could be seen. (From the patient, performing coal transportation for 25 years)

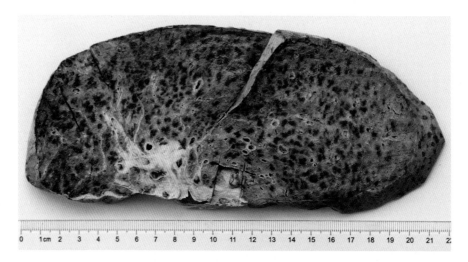

图 4　肺内煤斑灶：肺切面可见较多黑色斑灶样病变，肺门淋巴结肿大伴煤尘沉积。(采煤工作 26 年)

Fig.4　Pulmonary coal dust maculae: A large amount of black maculae are shown on the cut surface of the lung, with enlarged hilar lymph nodes and coal dust deposition. (From the patient, performing coal mining work for 26 years)

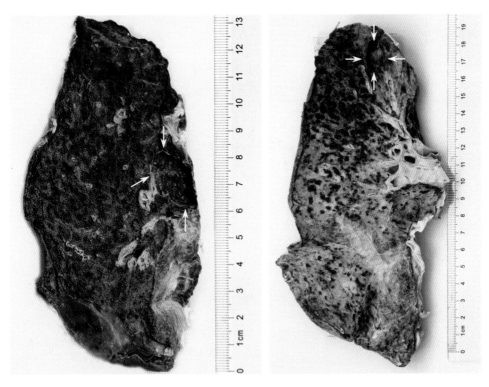

图 5　肺内煤斑灶伴大泡型肺气肿形成：肺切面可见黑色斑灶样病变，肺内大泡型肺气肿形成（箭头所指）。左图（掘进工作 20 年）；右图（采煤、通风工作 19 年）。

Fig.5　Pulmonary coal dust maculae accompanied by bullous emphysema: The black maculae are accompanied by bullous emphysema (white arrows).[From the patients, working in coal tunneling for 20 years (left), and coal mining and ventilation work for 19 years (right)].

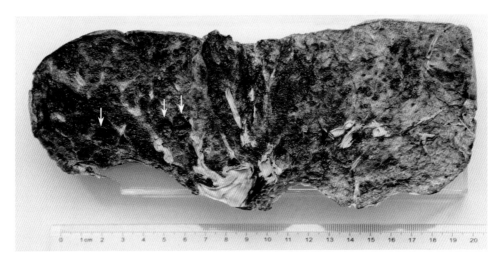

图 6　肺内煤斑灶伴囊泡型肺气肿形成：肺切面可见黑色斑灶样病变，伴有囊泡型肺气肿形成（箭头所指）。（掘进工作 17 年）

Fig.6　Pulmonary coal dust maculae with cystic emphysema: Black maculae are admixed in cystic emphysema (white arrows) on the cut surface of lung. (From the patient, working in coal tunneling for 17 years)

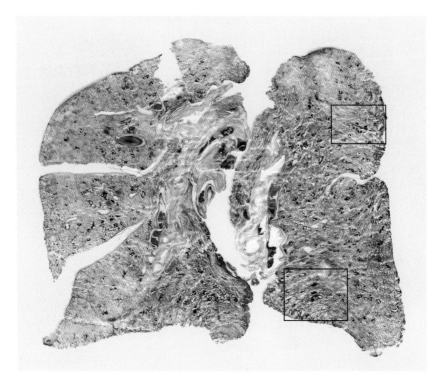

图 7　肺内煤斑灶（全肺大切片标本）:(厚 20μm）可见诸多黑色斑灶样病变,伴局部小气道扩张,肺门淋巴结肿大,煤尘沉积。(掘进、采煤工作 15 年）

Fig.7　Pulmonary coal dust maculae (the large slice): 20 μm in thickness, showing the sagittal section of the whole lung, demonstrates a variety of alterations in lung, including black coal dust maculae, partial dilated small airways, enlarged hilar lymph nodes and coal dust deposits. (From the patient, performing coal tunneling and mining works for 15 years)

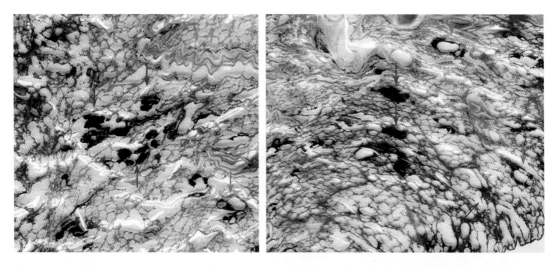

图 8　肺内煤斑灶（全肺大切片标本）（图 7 局部放大）:绿色箭头指尘斑（气肿）病变;红色箭头指尘灶病变。

Fig.8　Pulmonary coal dust maculae (the large slice) (regional amplification of Fig.7): Coal dust dots (around the emphysema sites, green arrows), consolidated coal dust foci (red arrows).

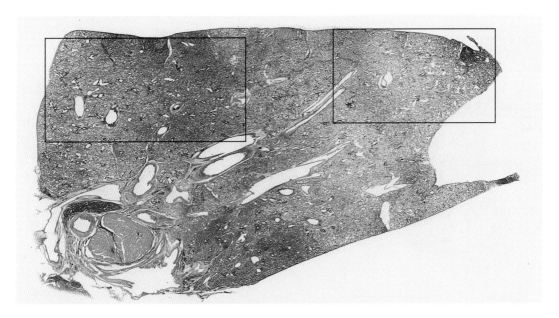

图 9　肺内煤斑灶 (肺叶大切片标本):可见一些黑色的斑灶样病变,局部有 1 个煤矽结节形成。(井下采煤等工作 24 年)

Fig.9　Pulmonary coal dust maculae: The large slice, showing cross-section of the whole pulmonary lobe, illustrates the formation of black coal dust maculae. Note a coal silicotic nodule is adjacent to the pleura. (From the patient, performing coal mining works for 24 years)

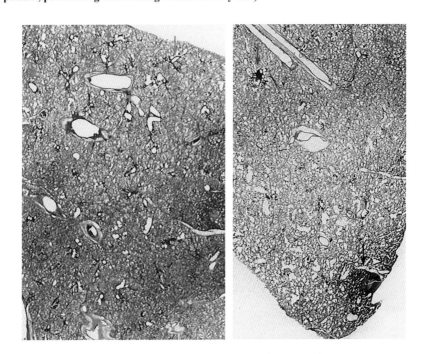

图 10　肺内煤斑灶 (全肺大切片标本)(图 9 局部放大):绿色箭头所指尘斑(气肿)病变;红色箭头所指煤尘灶病变,黑色箭头所指煤矽结节。

Fig.10　Pulmonary coal dust maculae (the large slice) (regional amplification of Fig.9): Coal dust dots (around the emphysema sites, green arrows), coal dust foci (red arrows), coal silicotic nodules (black arrows).

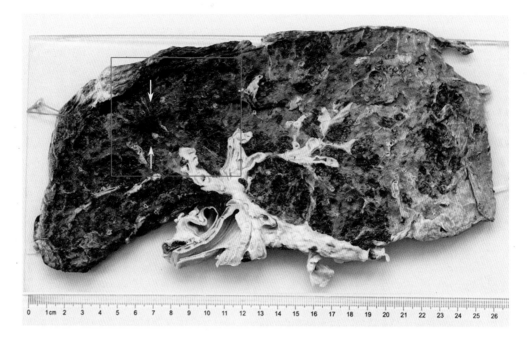

图 11　肺内煤斑灶、煤尘纤维灶（煤结节）形成:箭头所指黑色、质实、呈星芒状向四周伸延。(采煤工作 21 年)

Fig.11　Pulmonary coal dust maculae and fibrotic lesions (coal dust nodule): A stellate-shaped, consolidated, black coal dust fibrotic lesion (white arrows), spreads to the surrounding tissue. (From the patient, performing coal mining works for 21 years)

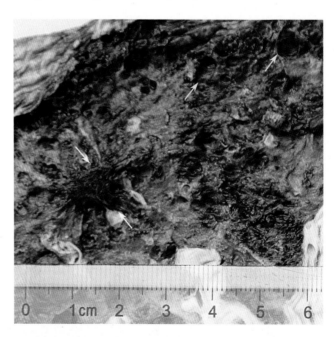

图 12　肺内煤斑灶、煤尘纤维灶（煤结节）形成（图 11 局部放大）:煤尘纤维灶(煤结节,直径达 1cm,白色箭头)、囊泡型肺气肿(黄色箭头)。

Fig.12　Pulmonary coal dust maculae and fibrotic lesions (coal dust nodule) (regional amplification of Fig.11): Coal dust fibrotic lesion (1cm in diameter, white arrows), cystic emphysemas (yellow arrows).

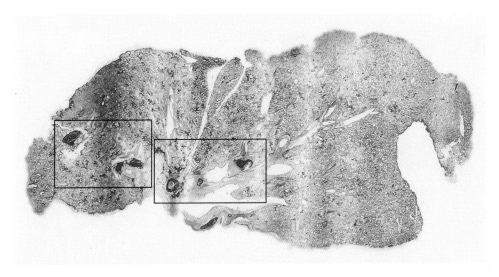

图 13 肺内煤斑灶、煤矽结节:左肺大切片标本,可见一些黑色斑灶样和结节病变。(采煤、掘进、井下运输工作 31 年)

Fig.13 Pulmonary coal dust maculae and coal silicotic nodules: The large slice shows sagittal section of whole left lung. Note the black coal dust maculae and the nodular lesions. (From the patient, working in coal mining, tunneling and transportation for 31 years)

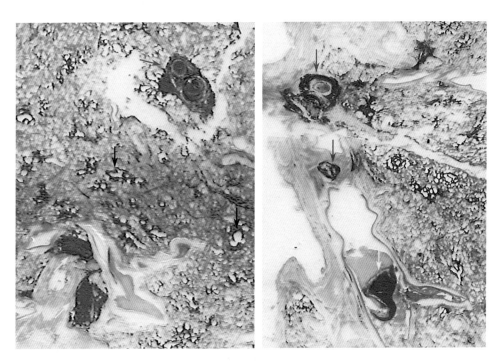

图 14 肺内煤斑灶、煤矽结节(图 13 局部放大):黑色箭头指尘斑(气肿)病变;绿色箭头指煤尘纤维灶病变,红色色箭头指煤矽结节,黄色箭头指肺内支气管旁淋巴结煤尘沉积。

Fig.14 Pulmonary coal dust maculae and coal silicotic nodules (regional amplification of Fig.13): Coal dust dots (around the emphysema sites, black arrows), coal silicotic lesions (green arrows), coal silicotic nodules (red arrows), and coal dust deposition in the paratracheal lymph node (yellow arrows).

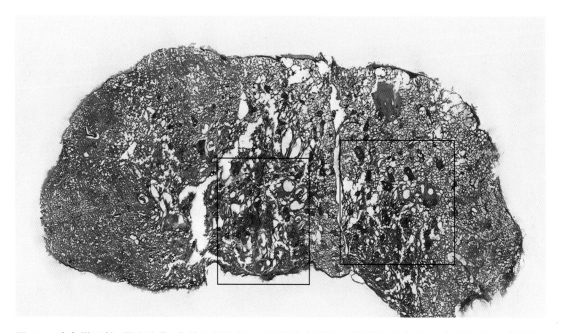

图 15　肺内煤斑灶、煤矽结节：右肺大切片标本，可见诸多黑色斑灶样和结节病变，伴局部小气道扩张。（掘进、钻岩工作 12 年）

Fig.15　Pulmonary coal dust maculae and coal silicotic nodules: The large slice shows sagittal section of the whole right lung. Note coal dust maculae and coal dust nodular lesions, and partial small airways dilation. (From the patient, performing coal tunneling and rock drilling work for 12 years)

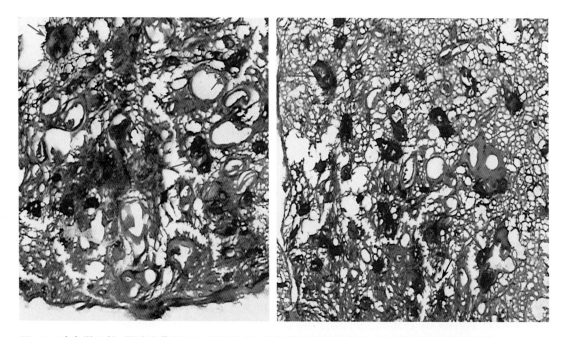

图 16　肺内煤斑灶、煤矽结节（图 15 局部放大）：绿色箭头所指煤尘灶、红色箭头所指煤矽结节。

Fig.16　Pulmonary coal dust maculae and coal silicotic nodules (regional amplification of Fig.15): Coal dust maculae (green arrows) and coal silicotic nodules (red arrows).

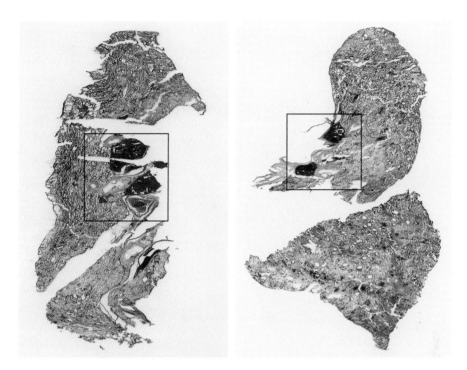

图 17 肺内煤斑灶:左、右肺大切片,肺内可见一些黑色斑灶样病变。肺门淋巴结肿大,伴煤尘沉积及煤矽结节形成。(采煤、掘进工作 29 年)

Fig.17 Pulmonary coal dust maculae: The large slices, showing sagittal section of the whole left lung and the whole right lung respectively, reveal the black coal dust maculae and the enlarged hilar lymph nodes, in response to coal dust deposits and coal silicotic nodule. (From the patient, working in coal mining and tunneling for 29 years)

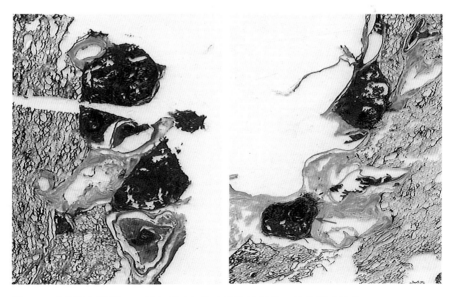

图 18 肺内煤斑灶(图 17 局部放大):箭头所指肺门淋巴结内煤矽结节。

Fig.18 Pulmonary coal dust maculae (regional amplification of Fig.17): Coal silicotic nodules in hilar lymph nodes (arrows).

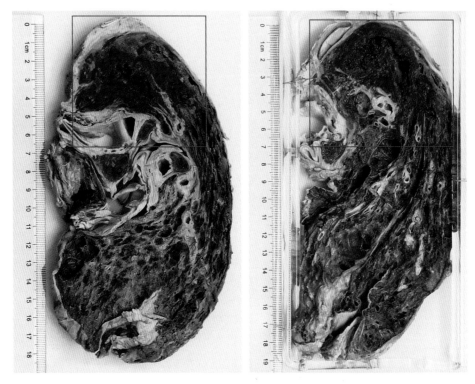

图 19　进行性块状纤维化(一个肺脏的两个切面):块状纤维化中裂隙样空洞形成。间质纤维化伴囊泡型、大泡型肺气肿、支气管扩张。胸膜增厚及血管内血栓形成。肺门淋巴结肿大伴煤尘沉积。(凿岩工作 20 年)

Fig.19　Progressive massive fibrosis: The bisected lung showing the slite-shaped cavities involved in the massive fibrotic lesions. It also illustrates other changes, including fibrosis reaction, cystic and bulbous emphysema of interstitial tissue, bronchiectasis, pleural thickening associated with intravascular thrombus, as well as enlarged hilar lymphatic nodes with coal dust deposition. (From the patient, performing coal rock drilling works for 20 years)

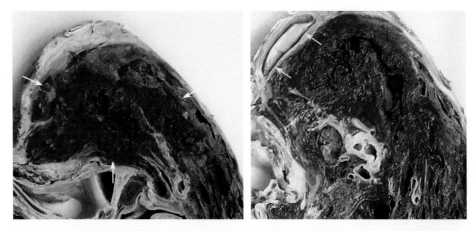

图 20　进行性块状纤维化(图 19 局部放大):进行性块状纤维化(白色箭头)、胸膜增厚(红色箭头)、血管内血栓形成(黄色箭头)。

Fig.20　Progressive massive fibrosis (regional amplification of Fig.19): Progressive massive fibrosis lesion (white arrows), pleura thickening (red arrow), intravascular thrombus (yellow arrow).

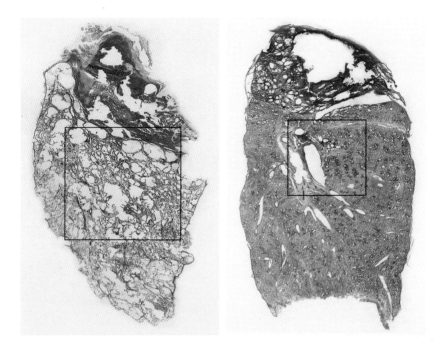

图21　进行性块状纤维化（肺大切片标本）：左、右肺上叶块状纤维化中组织坏死及空洞形成。左肺下叶肺间质纤维化及囊泡型及大泡型肺气肿形成。右肺下叶较多尘斑灶状病变，伴小支气管扩张。（左图，凿岩工作20年，右图掘进、井下运输工作22年）

Fig.21　Progressive massive fibrosis (the large slice): showing sagittal section of the whole left and right lung, reveal a wide variety of alterations of coal works' pneumoconiosis. ①Destruction of pulmonary tissue and necrotic cavities are formed in the massive fibrotic lesions, mainly located at the upper lobe of the left and right lung. ②The inferior lobe of the left lung shows fibrosis reaction, cystic and bullae emphysema in the interstitial tissue. ③A large amount of coal maculae could be seen in the inferior lobe of the right lung, with small bronchiole dilation.〔From the patients, performing coal rock drilling work for 20 years (left), or in coal tunneling and transportation for 22 years (right)〕

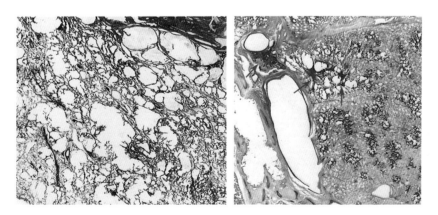

图22　进行性块状纤维化（肺大切片标本）（图21局部放大）：左图显示弥漫性间质纤维化伴囊泡型肺气肿。右图箭头所指煤尘纤维灶伴小叶中心型肺气肿。

Fig.22　Progressive massive fibrosi (the large slice) (regional amplification of Fig.21): The left photography illustration of diffuse interstitial fibrosis and cystic emphysema, and the right one showing coal dust fibrotic lesions, surrounding the centriacinar emphysema sites (red arrows).

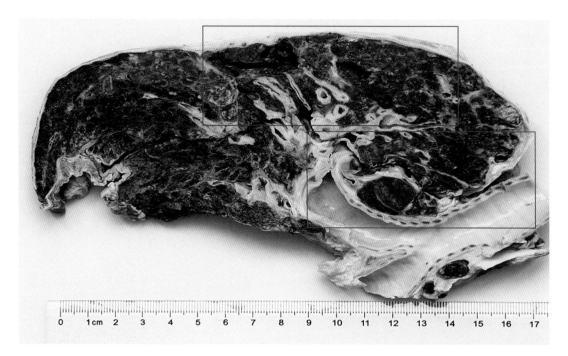

图 23　结节融合型块状纤维化：黑色、实性、块状（6cm×7cm）、质硬，可见诸多圆形煤矽结核结节融合在一起。肺内支气管扩张，胸膜增厚。肺门多个淋巴结肿大，煤尘沉积。（掘进、钻岩工作 12 年）

Fig.23　**Nodular confluent massive fibrosis: A large (6cm*7cm in area), consolidated, firm, black fibrotic lesion is present in lung, with the coalescence of many round coal silicotic tuberculous nodules. Meanwhile, bronchiectasis, pleural thickening and enlarged hilar lymph nodes with deposits of coal dust are all visible. (From the patient, performing coal tunneling and rock drilling work for 12 years)**

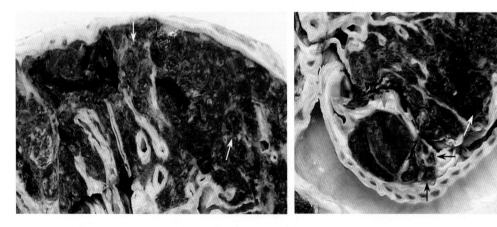

图 24　结节融合型块状纤维化（图 23 局部放大）：白色箭头显示融合型煤矽结核结节，红色箭头显示坏死性空洞，绿色箭头显示肿大的肺门淋巴结，黑色箭头显示淋巴结内融合型煤矽结核结节形成。

Fig.24　**Nodular confluent massive fibrosis (regional amplification of Fig.23): Confluent coal silicotic tuberculous nodules (white arrows), necrotic cavities (red arrows), enlarged hilar lymph nodes (green arrows), and confluent coal silicotic tuberculous nodules in lymph nodes (black arrows).**

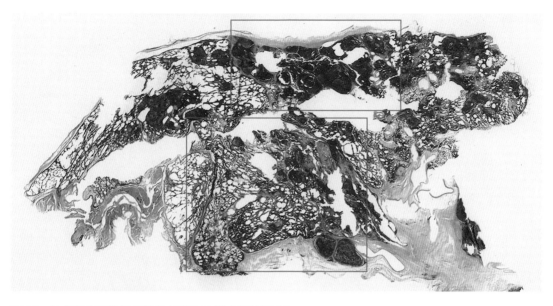

图25　结节融合型块状纤维化（同图23肺大切片标本）。

Fig.25　Nodular confluent massive fibrosis (this large slice shares the sample with Fig.23) .

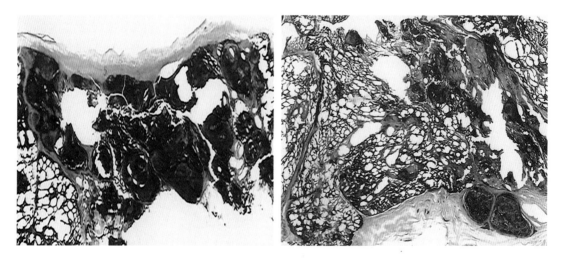

图26　结节融合型块状纤维化（图25局部放大）：左图显示肺内多数煤矽结核结节融合在一起，构成结节融合型块状纤维化。右图显示弥漫性间质纤维化伴肺气肿，肺门淋巴肿大及煤尘沉积。

Fig.26　Nodular confluent massive fibrosis (regional amplification of Fig.25: (Left) The production of nodular confluent massive fibrosis is created by the coalescence of numerous coal silicotic tuberculous nodules. (Right) The formation of diffusely scattered interstitial fibrosis reaction is associated with emphysema, enlarged hilar lymphatic nodes and coal dust deposits.

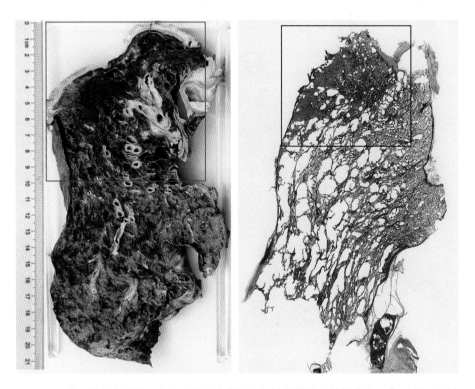

图 27　混合型块状纤维化：融合型煤矽结节与进行性纤维化斑块混杂在一起形成一团块病灶（黑色、实性、质硬，8cm×4cm），伴支气管扩张，胸膜增厚。（掘进工作 20 年）

Fig.27　Mixed massive fibrosis: A large (8cm*4cm in area), consolidated, firm, black fibrotic lesion is present in lung, with the fusion of confluent coal silicotic nodules and the progressive fibrotic plaques. Meanwhile, bronchiectasis and pleural thickening could be seen. (From the patient, working in coal tunneling for 20 years)

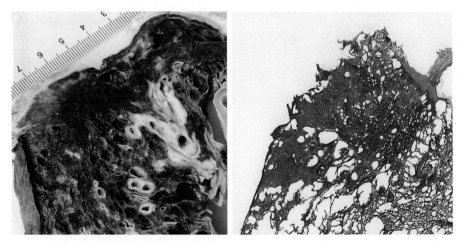

图 28　混合型块状纤维化（图 27 局部放大）：左图，绿色箭头为融合的结节病灶，红色箭头指块进行性状纤维化区域。右图，块状纤维化区域里煤尘沉积与纤维组织混杂在一起。

Fig.28　Mixed massive fibrosis (regional amplification of Fig.27): Confluent nodular lesions (green arrows, left) and progressive fibrotic lesions (red arrows, left). Coal dust deposits, admixed with proliferated fibrous tissue, are present in the massive fibrous lesion (Right).

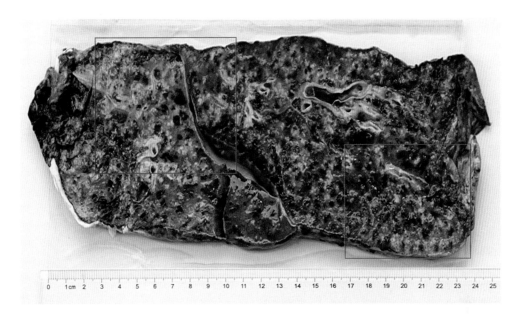

图 29 煤工尘肺伴结核病：肺内煤斑灶、播散性粟粒性肺结核及煤矽结核结节形成。（采煤工作 11 年）

Fig.29 Coal works' pneumoconiosis with tuberculosis: Coal dust maculae, disseminated miliary tuberculosis and coal silicotic tuberculous nodules are present in lung. (From the patient, performing coal mining works for 11 years)

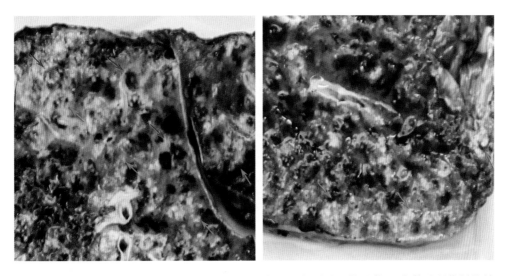

图 30 煤工尘肺伴结核病（图 29 局部放大）：红色箭头所指煤矽结核结节，绿色箭头所指播散性粟粒性结核病灶。

Fig.30 Coal works' pneumoconiosis with tuberculosis (regional amplification of Fig.29): Coal silicotic tuberculous nodules (red arrows) and disseminated miliary tuberculosis (green arrows).

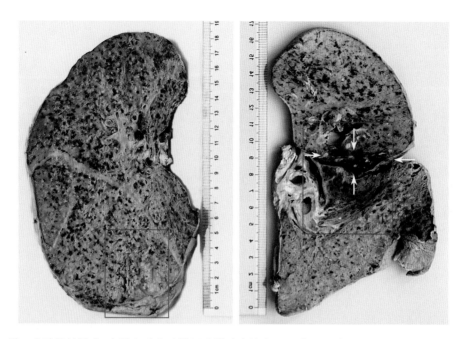

图 31 煤工尘肺伴结核病:左肺上叶大叶性干酪性肺炎伴空洞形成。近叶间裂处有一黑色纤维斑块形成(4cm×2cm,白色箭头所指),其内有数个白色斑点(结核病灶)。下叶近叶间裂处肺组织纤维化明显。右肺及左肺下叶密布粟粒性结核播散病灶。(井下机电维修工作 20 年)

Fig.31 Coal works' pneumoconiosis with tuberculosis: In the upper lobe of the left lung, caseous pneumonia is accompanied by the necrotic cavities, and a large area (4cm*2cm in area) of black fibrous lesion (white arrows), adjacent to the interlobar fissure, contains several white tuberculosis sites. In the inferior lobe of left lung, the pulmonary tissue close to the interlobar fissure is marked by dense collagen. Miliary tuberculosis is also widely distributed in both right lung and inferior lobe of left lung. (From the patient, working in underground maintenance of equipment and electricity for 20 years)

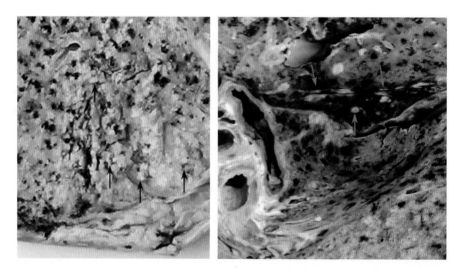

图 32 煤工尘肺伴结核病(图 31 局部放大):黑色箭头指粟粒性结核病灶,绿色箭头指块状纤维化内结核病灶。

Fig.32 Coal works' pneumoconiosis with tuberculosis (regional amplification of Fig.31): Miliary tuberculosis lesions (black arrows) and tuberculosis sites in the massive fibrosis lesion (green arrows).

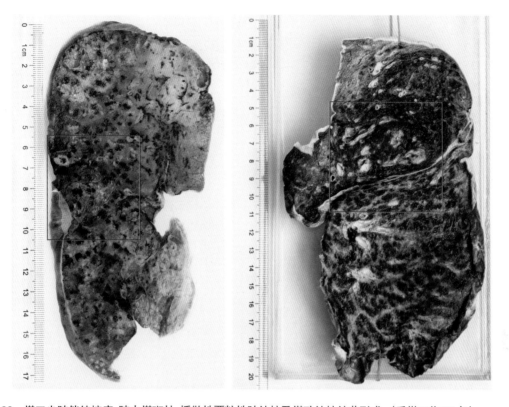

图 33　煤工尘肺伴结核病:肺内煤斑灶、播散性粟粒性肺结核及煤矽结核结节形成。(采煤工作 25 年)

Fig.33　Coal works' pneumoconiosis with tuberculosis: Pulmonary coal dust maculae, disseminated miliary tuberculosis and coal silicotic tuberculous nodules could be seen in lung. (From the patient, performing coal mining work for 25 years)

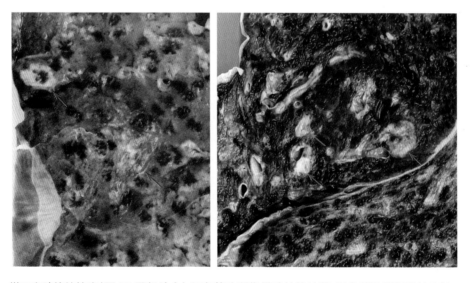

图 34　煤工尘肺伴结核病(图 33 局部放大):红色箭头所指煤矽结核结节,绿色箭头所指结核病灶。

Fig.34　Coal works' pneumoconiosis with tuberculosis (regional amplification of Fig.33): Coal silicotic tuberculous nodules (red arrows) and tuberculosis sites (green arrows).

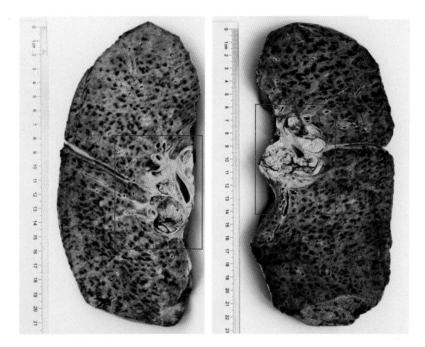

图 35　煤工尘肺伴结核病:肺内煤斑灶,肺门淋巴结肿大伴煤尘沉积及干酪样坏死病变。(掘进、采煤工作 20 年)

Fig.35　Coal works' pneumoconiosis with tuberculosis: Pulmonary coal dust maculae, enlarged hilar lymph nodes with coal dust deposition and caseous necrosis could be seen. (From the patient, performing coal tunneling and mining work for 20 years)

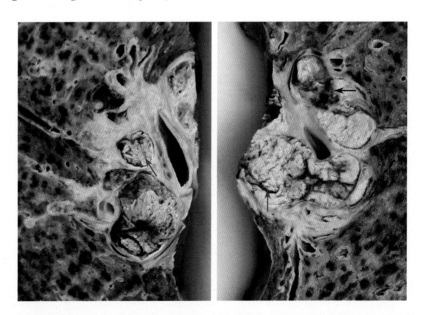

图 36　煤工尘肺伴结核病(图 35 局部放大):绿色箭头指淋巴结内煤矽结核结节形成。黑色箭头指淋巴结内煤尘沉积及尘性间质纤维化,红色箭头指结核性干酪样坏死。

Fig.36　Coal works' pneumoconiosis with tuberculosis (regional amplification of Fig.35): Coal silicotic tuberculous nodules in lymph nodes (green arrows), deposits of coal dust in fibrotic lymph nodes (black arrows), caseous necrosis (red arrows).

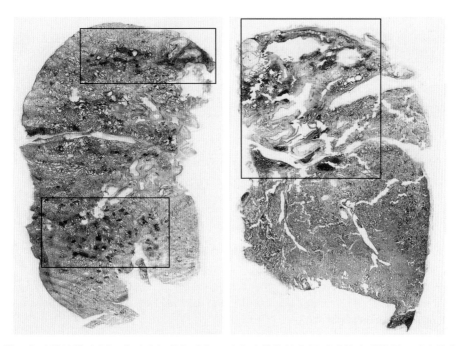

图 37 煤工尘肺伴结核病(左、右肺大切片标本):两肺上叶结核性空洞形成伴胸膜增厚。肺内诸多黑色斑灶样和结节病变分布,伴局部小气道扩张。(掘进、运输工作 22 年)

Fig.37 Coal works' pneumoconiosis with tuberculosis: The large slices, showing sagittal sections of the whole left and right lung. Note tuberculous cavities and thickened pleura in the superior lobes, with scattered coal maculae and nodular lesions, dilatated small airway. (From the patient, performing coal tunneling and transportation for 22 years)

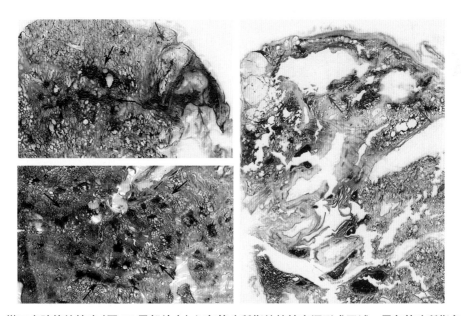

图 38 煤工尘肺伴结核病(图 37 局部放大):红色箭头所指结核性空洞形成区域。黑色箭头所指多数煤矽结节形成区域。

Fig.38 Coal works' pneumoconiosis with tuberculosis (regional amplification of Fig.37): Tuberculous cavities (red arrows), coal silicotic nodules (black arrows).

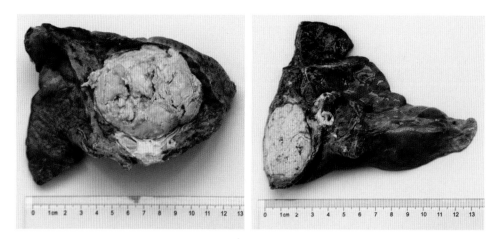

图 39　煤工尘肺伴肺癌（周围型）:煤尘沉积肺叶的切面可见一个类圆形灰黄色的癌结节。（掘进工作 20 年）

Fig.39　Coal works' pneumoconiosis with lung cancer (Peripheral type): A round, well demarcated, gray-yellow tumor mass in the coal dust-deposited lobe. (From the patient, working in coal tunneling for 20 years)

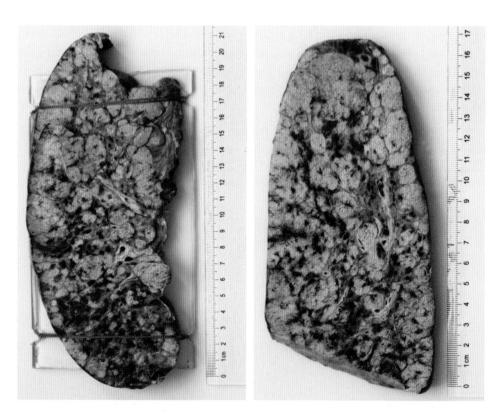

图 40　煤工尘肺伴肺癌（弥漫型）:煤尘沉积的肺叶内弥漫遍布大小不等灰黄色的癌结节。（掘进、采煤工作 25 年）

Fig.40　Coal works' pneumoconiosis with lung cancer (Diffuse type): Cross-section of coal dust-deposited lung evidence of multiple widespread tumor masses, characterized by gray yellow color and different size. (From the patient, performing coal tunneling and mining work for 25 years)

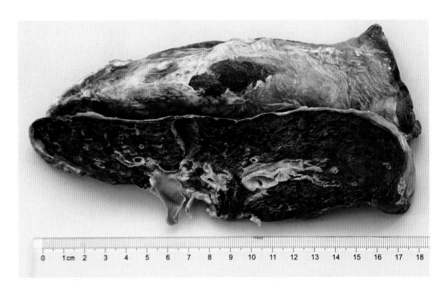

图 41 煤工尘肺伴胸膜粘连与增厚。(掘进、采煤工作 23 年)

Fig.41 Coal works' pneumoconiosis with pleural adhesion and thickening. (From the patient, working in coal tunneling and mining for 23 years)

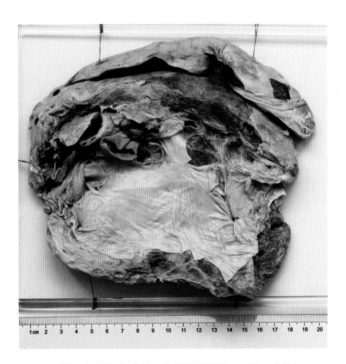

图 42 煤工尘肺伴胸膜粘连与增厚（与图 41 同一病例）。

Fig.42 Coal works' pneumoconiosis with pleural adhesion and thickening (sample is same as Fig.41).

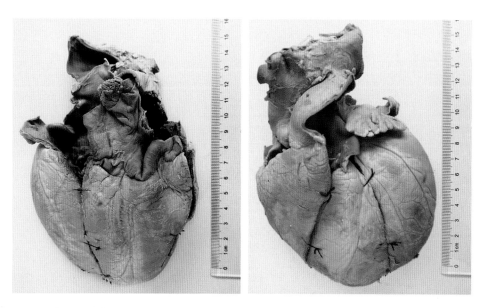

图43 煤工尘肺合并肺源性心脏病:心脏体积增大,重量增加(350g),心尖钝圆。心脏呈顺时针方向转位,心脏前壁由左心室与右心室共同构成,整个心脏呈球形外观(左图:心脏正面;右图:心脏背面)。(井下采煤、通风工作19年)

Fig.43 Coal works' pneumoconiosis with cor pulmonale: The heart has increased mass and weight (350g), with blunt apex. The ball heart takes a clockwise rotation, the anterior wall consisting of right ventricle and left ventricle. (Left: anterior heart, right: posterior heart). (From the patient, working coal mining and ventilation for 19 years)

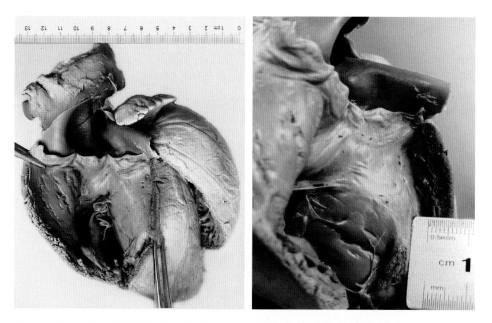

图44 煤工尘肺合并肺源性心脏病:右心室腔扩张,右心室壁增厚(超过5mm)(与图43同一心脏)。

Fig.44 Coal works' pneumoconiosis with cor pulmonale: Right ventricular dilation with thickened ventricular wall (more than 5mm in thickness). (Sample is same as Fig.43)

第二部分
煤工尘肺组织形态学特点

Part II
Histological Appearance of Coal Workers' Pneumoconiosis

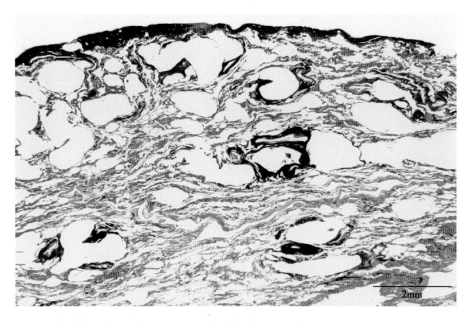

图 45 胸膜煤斑:较多煤尘沉积在胸膜,胸膜增厚。胸膜下方肺泡腔扩张、肺气肿形成。(采煤、掘进工作 11 年)(H.E 染色)

Fig.45 Coal dust dots of pleura: Coal dust deposits thicken the pleura mildly, with subpleural emphysema characterized by airspaces enlargement. (From the patient, working in coal mining and tunneling for 11 years) (H.E stain)

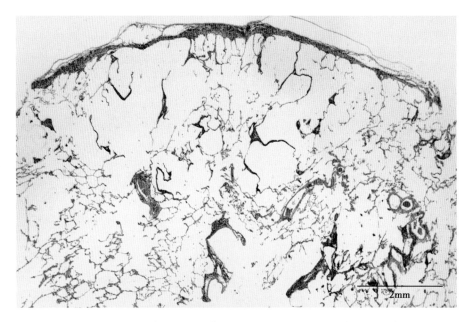

图 46 胸膜煤斑:大量煤尘沉积在胸膜,伴有少量纤维组织增生,胸膜增厚。胸膜下方肺泡腔扩张、肺气肿形成。(采煤、通风工作 22 年)(H.E 染色)

Fig.46 Coal dust dots of pleura: Deposits of coal dust and mild fibrous proliferation thicken the regional pleura. Note subpleural emphysema, showing marked enlargement of airspaces. (From the patient, working in coal mining and ventilation for 22 years) (H.E stain)

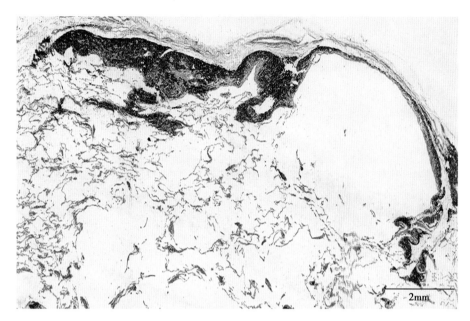

图 47　胸膜煤斑：大量煤尘沉积在胸膜伴纤维组织增生、胸膜增厚。煤斑一侧肺泡腔高度扩张。(采煤、掘进工作 11 年)(H.E 染色)

Fig.47　Coal dust dots of pleura: Deposits of coal dust and mild fibrous proliferation thicken the regional pleura. Note a highly expansive airspace at one side of coal dust dot. (From the patient, working in coal mining and tunneling for 11 years) (H.E stain)

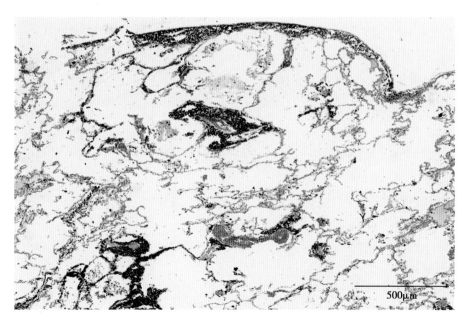

图 48　胸膜煤斑：较多的煤尘沉积在胸膜，胸膜增厚。胸膜下方肺组织内小血管周围粉尘沉积，伴部分肺泡腔扩张。(采煤、掘进工作 21 年)(H.E 染色)

Fig.48　Coal dust dots of pleura: Microscopic view shows moderate amount of coal dust deposits either in pleura or around subpleural small blood vessels, causing pleural thickening and surrounding airspaces enlarging. (From the patient, working in coal mining and tunneling for 21 years) (H.E stain)

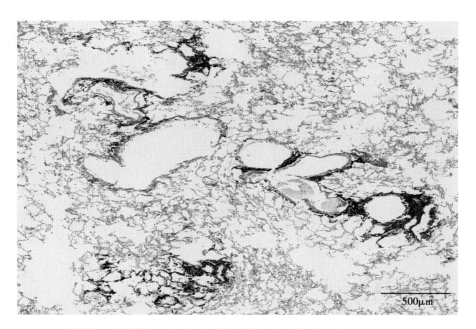

图 49　肺内煤斑:少量煤尘沉积在呼吸性支气管、肺泡管、肺泡囊及小血管周围,伴肺泡道和肺泡腔扩张。(掘进、回采工作 15 年)(H.E 染色)

Fig.49　Coal dust dots of lung: Minimal coal dust deposits around the respiratory bronchia, alveolar ducts, alveolar sacs and small vessels, with expansion of respiratory units. (From the patient, working in coal tunneling and mining for 15 years) (H.E stain)

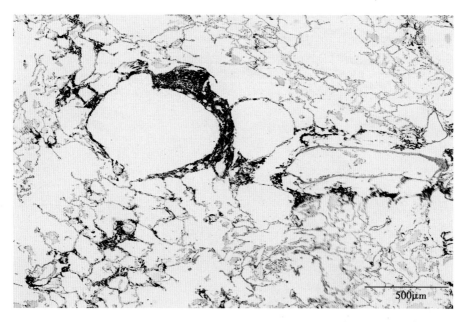

图 50　肺内煤斑:少量煤尘沉积在呼吸性支气管、肺泡管及肺泡囊周围,伴肺泡腔扩张。(采煤工作 17 年)(H.E 染色)

Fig.50　Coal dust dots of lung: Minimal coal dust deposits around the respiratory bronchi, alveolar ducts and alveolar sacs, with marked enlargement of airspaces. (From the patient, working in coal mining for 17 years) (H.E stain)

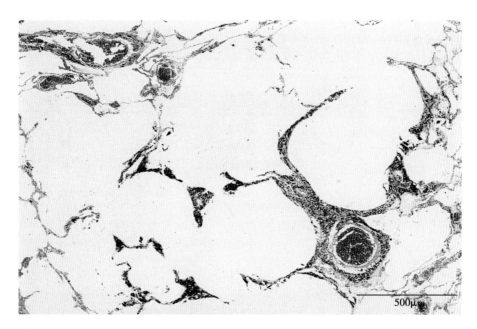

图51　肺内煤斑:煤尘沉积在肺泡管及肺泡囊及小血管周围,伴肺泡道、肺泡腔扩张。(采煤、掘进工作 17 年)(H.E 染色)

Fig.51　Coal dust dots of lung: Coal dust deposits around alveolar ducts, alveolar sacs and small vessels, with enlargement of the surrounding respiratory units. (From the patient, working in coal mining and tunneling for 17 years) (H.E stain)

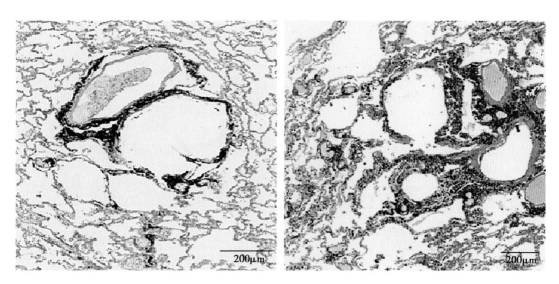

图 52　肺内煤斑:少量煤尘沉积在呼吸性细支气管、肺泡管及小血管周围,伴呼吸性细支气管和肺泡腔扩张。(掘进、回采工作 15 年)(H.E 染色)

Fig.52　Coal dust dots of lung: Minimal coal dust deposition around respiratory bronchia, alveolar ducts and small blood vessels, with marked enlargement of respiratory bronchia and alveolar spaces. (From the patient, working in coal tunneling and mining for 15 years) (H.E stain)

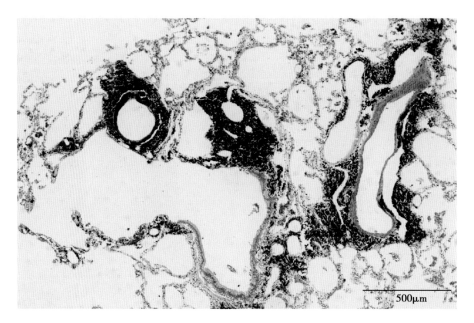

图 53　煤尘细胞灶:较多煤尘沉积在呼吸性细支气管和小血管周围,在呼吸性细支气管形成两个实性煤尘细胞灶,呼吸性细支气管扩张。(掘进、回采工作 17 年)(H.E 染色)

Fig.53　Cellular coal dust foci: Large amount of coal dust deposits around the respiratory bronchia may facilitate to form two consolidated black cellular lesions, with dilation of the surrounding respiratory bronchia. Same response is also seen at the site of small blood vessels. (From the patient, working in coal tunneling and mining for 17 years) (H.E stain)

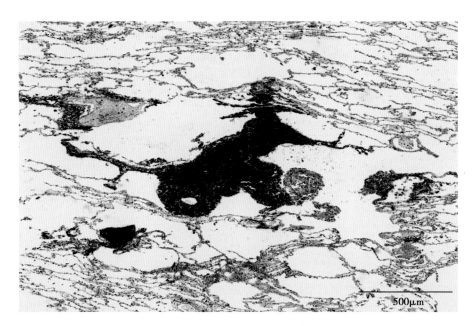

图 54　煤尘细胞灶:煤尘沉积形成实性细胞灶,呼吸性细支气管扩张。(掘进工作 17 年)(H.E 染色)

Fig.54　Cellular coal dust foci: A consolidated black area represents cellular coal dust focus due to coal dust deposition, with dilation of the surrounding respiratory bronchia. (From the patient, working in coal tunneling for 17 years) (H.E stain)

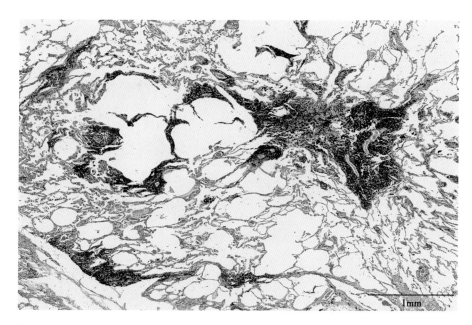

图 55　煤尘纤维灶:较多煤尘沉积在呼吸性细支气管、肺泡管及肺泡囊周围,局部形成实性多脚状病灶向外伸延,病灶内一定量胶原沉积,伴全小叶型肺气肿形成。(掘进工作 20 年)(H.E 染色)

Fig.55　Fibrous coal dust foci: A moderate amount of coal dust deposits around respiratory bronchia, alveolar ducts, and alveolar sacs. In a patchy area, coal dust deposits and the proliferated fibrous tissue create a star-shaped consolidated lesion, spreading to the surrounding tissue. Panacinar emphysema is visible. (From the patient, working in coal tunneling for 20 years) (H.E tain)

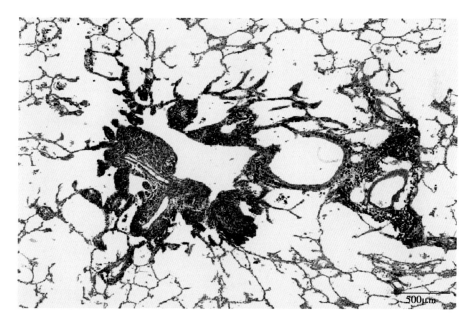

图 56　煤尘纤维灶:较大的煤尘纤维灶形成,并呈放射状向四周伸延,呼吸性细支气管扩张。(采煤、掘进工作 11 年)(H.E 染色)

Fig.56　Fibrous coal dust foci: The photography shows a larger star-shaped coal dust fibrous focus, extending to the surrounding tissue, with focal respiratory bronchia dilation. (From the patient, working in coal mining and tunneling for 11 years) (H.E stain)

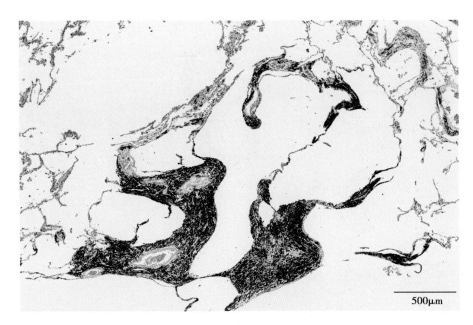

图 57　煤尘纤维灶:两个煤尘纤维灶沉积在呼吸性细支气管壁两侧,伴全小叶型肺气肿形成。(采煤、通风工作 22 年)(H.E 染色)

Fig.57　Fibrous coal dust foci: The respiratory bronchial wall has been sectioned to reveal the two symmetrical fibrous coal dust foci, surrounded by alterations of panacinar emphysema. (From the patient, working in coal mining and ventilation for 22 years) (H.E stain)

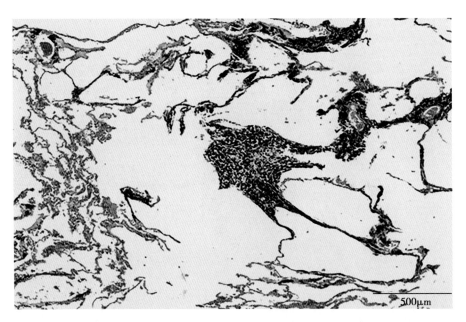

图 58　煤尘纤维灶:煤尘纤维灶突入呼吸性细支气管,伴全小叶型肺气肿形成。(采煤、通风工作 22 年)(H.E 染色)

Fig.58　Fibrous coal dust foci: Microscopic view illustrates a fibrous coal dust focus is projecting into the lumen of respiratory bronchiole. Panacinar emphysema is seen. (From the patient, working in coal mining and ventilation for 22 years) (H.E stain)

图 59 至图 74 大小不等、形状各异的煤尘灶
Fig.59 to Fig.74 Coal dust lesions varying in size and shape

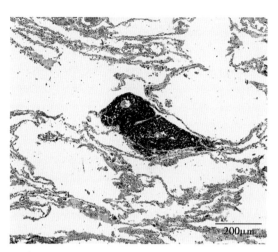

图 59　云雀状（H.E 染色）

Fig.59　Skylark like coal dust lesion (H.E stain)

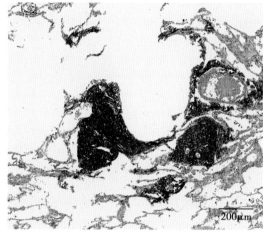

图 60　信鸽状（H.E 染色）

Fig.60　Pigeon like coal dust lesion (H.E stain)

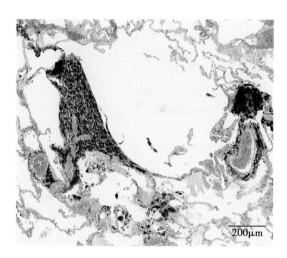

图 61　啄木鸟状（H.E 染色）

Fig.61　Woodpecker like coal dust lesion (H.E stain)

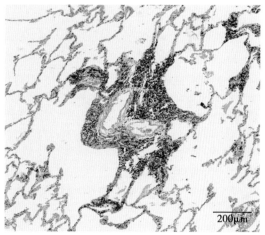

图 62　鹭鸶状（H.E 染色）

Fig.62　Egret like coal dust lesion (H.E stain)

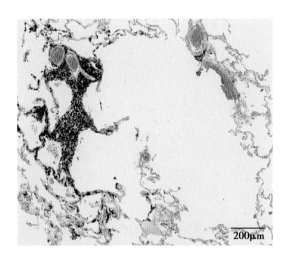

图 63　米老鼠状（H.E 染色）

Fig.63　Mickey mouse like coal dust lesion (H.E stain)

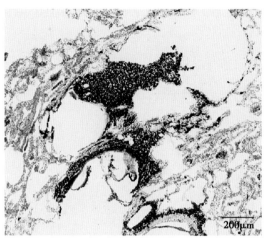

图 64　玩具熊状（H.E 染色）

Fig.64　Teddy bear like coal dust lesion (H.E stain)

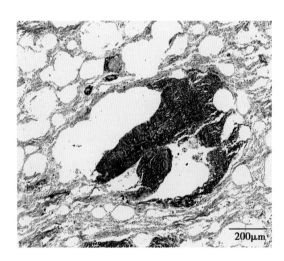

图 65　运动健将状（H.E 染色）

Fig.65　Sportsman like coal dust lesion (H.E stain)

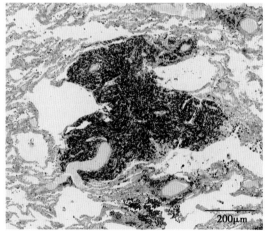

图 66　玉兔状（H.E 染色）

Fig.66　Rabbit like coal dust lesion (H.E stain)

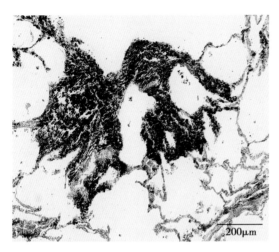

图 67 彩蝶状（H.E 染色）
Fig.67 Butterfly like coal dust lesion (H.E stain)

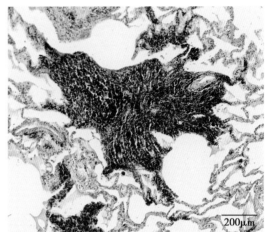

图 68 碟筝状（H.E 染色）
Fig.68 Butterfly kite like coal dust lesion (H.E stain)

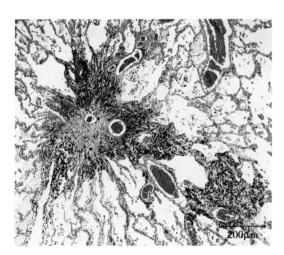

图 69 星芒状（H.E 染色）
Fig.69 Starry like coal dust lesion (H.E stain)

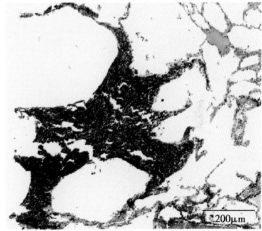

图 70 海星状（H.E 染色）
Fig.70 Starfish like coal dust lesion (H.E stain)

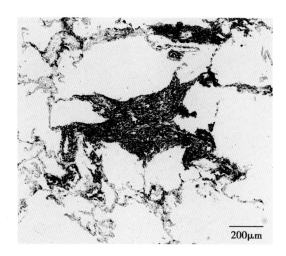

图 71 海蟹状（H.E 染色）
Fig.71 Sea crab like coal dust lesion (H.E stain)

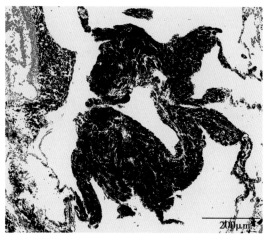

图 72 领结状（H.E 染色）
Fig.72 Bow-tie like coal dust lesion (H.E stain)

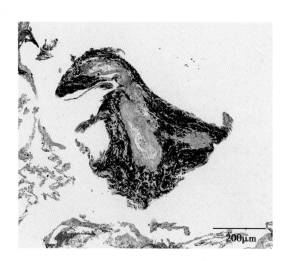

图 73 企鹅状（H.E 染色）
Fig.73 Unicorn like coal dust lesion (H.E stain)

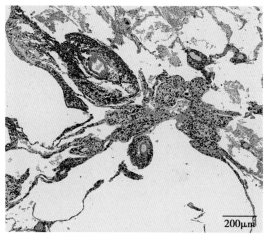

图 74 "敦煌壁画 - 飞天状"（H.E 染色）
Fig.74 Coal dust lesion resemble the flying fairy from Dunhuang Mural. (H.E stain)

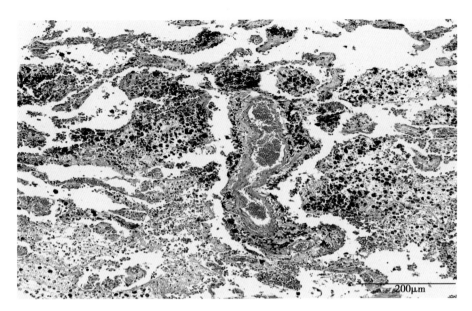

图 75　巨噬细胞性肺泡炎：吞噬煤尘的巨噬细胞（煤尘细胞）充填在肺泡腔与小血管周围伴其它炎细胞浸润。肺间质小血管与肺泡隔内毛细血管扩张充血。（采煤、掘进工作 11 年）（H.E 染色）

Fig.75　Macrophage alveolitis: Low-power view shows numerous coal dust-laden macrophages, predominantly fill in the alveolar spaces or around small blood vessels, associated with occasional other inflammatory cells. Congestion response occurs in the small blood vessels and capillaries of the alveolar septum. (From the patient, working in coal mining and tunneling for 11 years) (H.E stain)

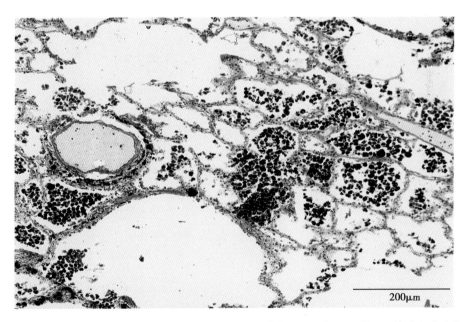

图 76　巨噬细胞性肺泡炎：较多吞噬煤尘巨噬细胞聚集充填在肺泡腔与小血管周。终末细小支气管和肺泡腔扩张。（井下测量工作 15 年）（H.E 染色）

Fig.76　Macrophage alveolitis: Abundant coal dust-laden macrophages aggregation in the alveolar space or around some small blood vessels, with expansion of terminal bronchia and alveolar spaces. (From the patient, performing underground survey working for 15 years) (H.E stain)

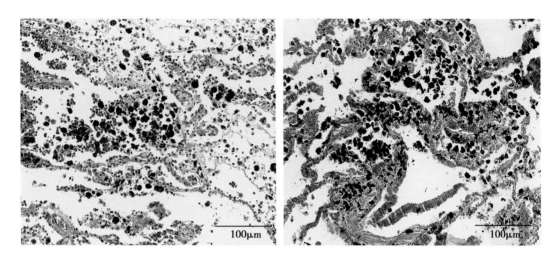

图 77　巨噬细胞性肺泡炎：肺泡腔内吞噬煤尘巨噬细胞聚集伴其他炎细胞浸润。肺泡隔内毛细血管扩张充血。（采煤、掘进工作 11 年）（H.E 染色）

Fig.77　Macrophage alveolitis: Numerous coal dust-laden macrophages and occasional other inflammatory cells are visible in the alveolar space. Capillaries of alveolar septum are congestion. (From the patient, working in coal mining and tunneling for 11 years) (H.E stain)

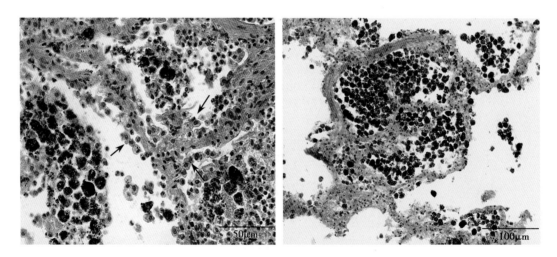

图 78　巨噬细胞性肺泡炎：吞噬煤尘巨噬细胞聚集充填在肺泡腔，伴其他炎细胞浸润及肺泡壁纤维组织增生。左图显示伴有肺泡壁 II 型上皮细胞增生（箭头所指），右图显示向早期煤尘细胞性结节的过度。（掘进、采煤工作 15 年）（H.E 染色）

Fig.78　Macrophage alveolitis: Coal dust-laden macrophages predominant inflammation in the alveolar spaces, with other inflammatory cells and dense collagen of alveolar wall. The proliferated type II alveolar cells are denoted by arrows of the left photography. These alterations may be regarded as the basis of cellular coal dust nodules as evidenced by the right one. (From the patient, working in coal tunneling and mining for 15 years) (H.E stain)

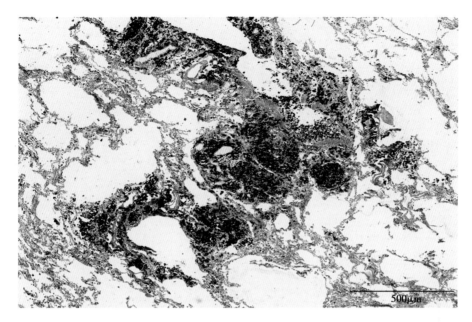

图 79 煤尘细胞性结节：较多煤尘聚集在肺泡腔，局部形成多个圆形、类圆结节状病灶，可伴有肺泡腔的轻度扩张。（掘进、采煤工作 15 年）（H.E 染色）

Fig.79 Cellular coal dust nodules: Cells with coal dust aggregate in the alveolar spaces, forming multiple round or quasi-circular nodules, with mild expansion of alveolar space. (From the patient, working in coal tunneling and mining for 15 years) (H.E stain)

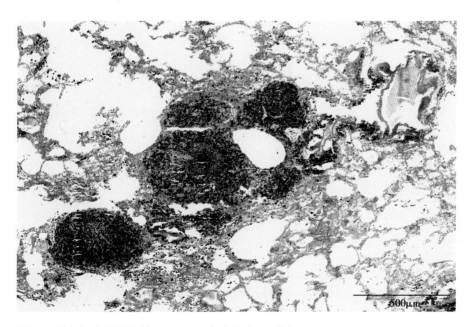

图 80 煤尘细胞性结节（与图 79 同一标本）。（H.E 染色）

Fig.80 Cellular coal dust nodules (sample is same as Fig. 79). (H.E stain)

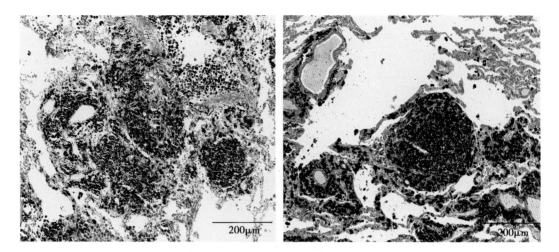

图 81　煤尘细胞性结节:左图显示多个煤尘细胞性结节形成,间质纤维组织增生,肺泡隔增宽。右图显示煤尘细胞性结节突入终末细支气管腔,伴小气道的扩张。(掘进、采煤工作 15 年)(H.E 染色)

Fig.81　Cellular coal dust nodules: The left photography illustrates multiple cellular coal dust nodules in lung, with dense collagen of interstitial tissue and thickening of alveolar septum, while the right one shows a cellular coal dust nodule projecting into the lumen of terminal respiratory bronchiole, with dilatation of the small airways. (From the patient, working in coal tunneling and mining for 15 years) (H.E stain)

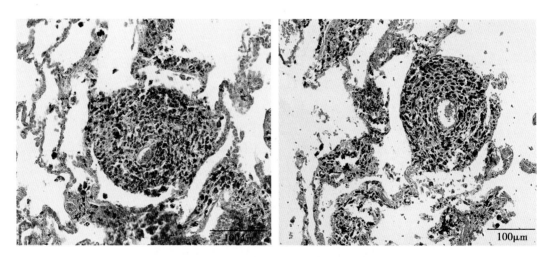

图 82　煤尘细胞性结节:煤尘细胞性结节内可见扩张充血的小血管。(左图井下测量工作 15 年,右图掘进、采煤工作 17 年)(H.E 染色)

Fig.82　Cellular coal dust nodules: The congested blood vessel could be seen in a cellular coal dust nodule.〔From the patients, performing underground survey works for 15 years (left), and working in coal tunneling and mining for 17 years (right)〕(H.E stain)

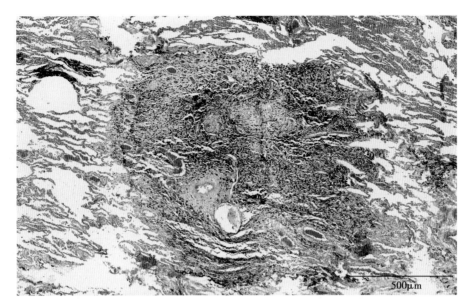

图 83 细胞纤维性结节（较大细胞纤维性结节）:结节内较多煤尘沉积伴胶原纤维增生及小血管增生充血,可见多个小结节融合的迹象。(掘进工作 20 年)（H.E 染色）

Fig.83 Cellular fibrous nodules: Several small cellular nodules show the tendency of fusion, forming a larger nodule containing coal dust deposits, modest amount of collagen fibers, and congested small blood vessels. (From the patient, working in coal tunneling for 20 years) (H.E stain)

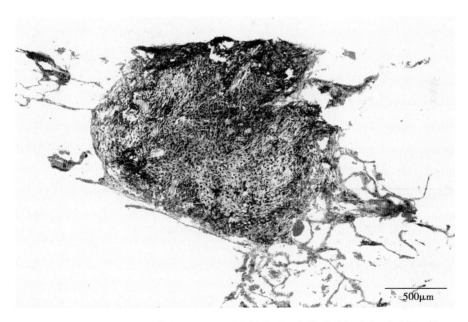

图 84 细胞纤维性结节:结节内煤尘沉积伴有较多胶原纤维增生与分布。(采煤工作 26 年)（H.E 染色）

Fig.84 Cellular fibrous nodules: The nodule in photography containing numerous deposits of coal dust and dense collagen. (From the patient, performing coal mining works for 26 years) (H.E stain)

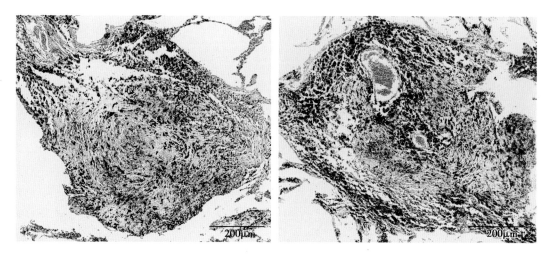

图 85　细胞纤维性结节：结节内煤尘沉积伴胶原纤维增生及小血管增生充血。（掘进工作 20 年）（H.E 染色）

Fig.85　Cellular fibrous nodules: Abundant coal dust deposits and dense collagen in the cellular fibrous nodules. (From the patient, working in coal tunneling for 20 years) (H.E stain)

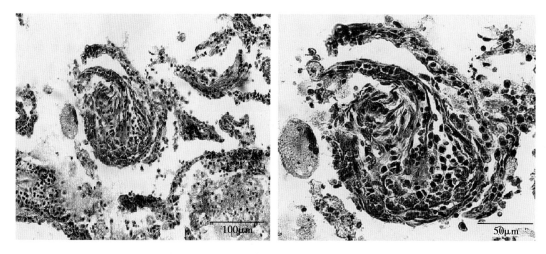

图 86　细胞纤维性结节：右图为左图的放大。蓝色为分布在结节内的胶原纤维。（掘进工作 20 年）（Masson 染色）

Fig.86　Cellular fibrous nodules: Right photography shows high-power details of the cellular fibrous nodule. Collagen is stained with blue color. (From the patient, working in coal tunneling for 20 years) (Masson stain)

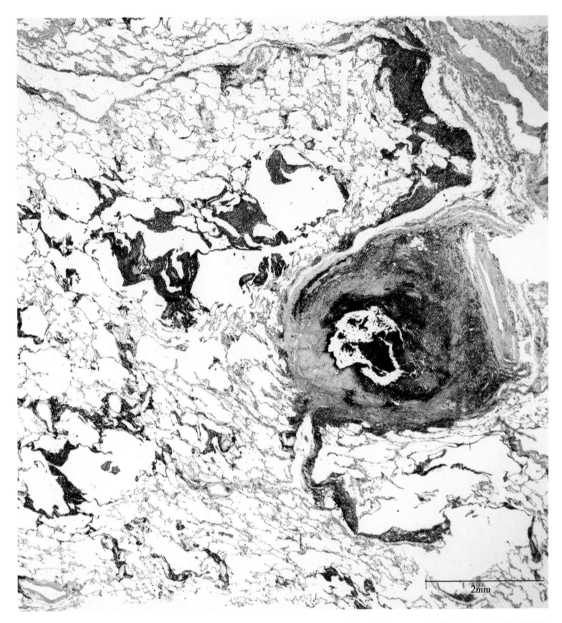

2mm

图 87 煤矽结节(纤维性结节):肺内较大结节病灶。结节内大量胶原纤维呈同心圆样分布,大量煤尘沉积在结节中央,形成煤尘池伴有组织的坏死。邻近肺组织内多个煤尘灶伴肺气肿形成。(井下采煤工作 8 年,井上其他混合工作 8 年)(H.E 染色)

Fig.87 Coal silicotic nodules (fibrous nodules): In lung, a larger coal silicotic nodule shows central coal dust deposits that may develop to "coal dust pool", tissue debris, and a peripheral accumulation of collagen arranged in a laminated pattern. Coal dust foci and emphysema sites are present in the surrounding tissue. (From the patient, working in coal mining and ground service for 8 years respectively) (H.E stain)

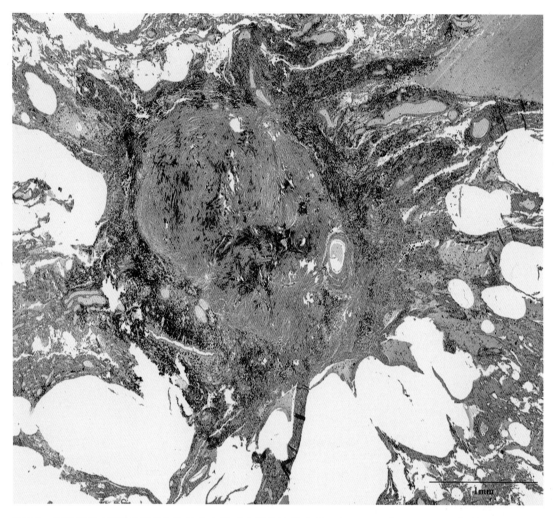

图 88　煤矽结节（纤维性结节）：结节内大量玻璃样变性的胶原沉积。可见煤尘沉积在结节外侧带呈"套袖样"结构。纤维性"毛发样伪足"向周边伸延。（掘进、采煤工作 26 年）（H.E 染色）

Fig.88　Coal silicotic nodules (fibrous nodules): Heavily deposited collagen fibers in the nodule occur to hyaline change, and coal dust deposits border the periphery of the lesion, looking like a "cuff-cover". The fibrous tissue protrudes from the lesion and extends toward the surrounding tissue, forming many hair shaped pseudopodia. (From the patient, performing in coal tunneling and mining for 26 years) (H.E stain)

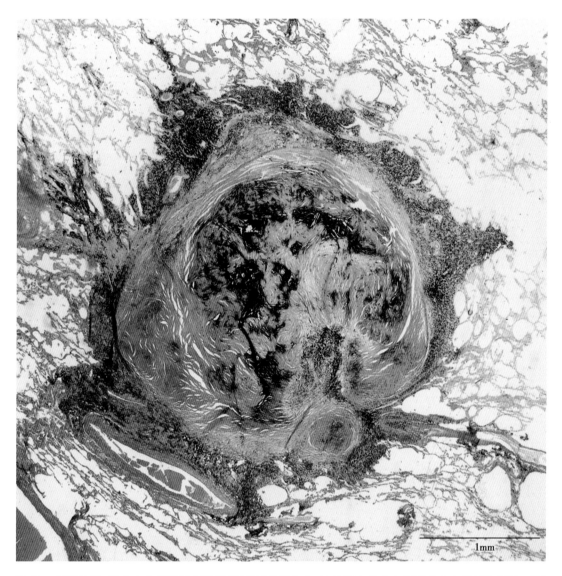

1mm

图89　煤矽结节：结节内大量胶原纤维呈"洋葱皮"样分布，较多煤尘分布在结节的中央区与外侧带。(采煤、掘进工作29年)(H.E染色)

Fig.89　Coal silicotic nodule: Heavily deposited collagen fibers in the nodule are noted as the pink laminated appearance, and a modest amount of coal dust deposits in the center of lesion and outside. (From the patient, performing on coal mining and tunneling for 29 years) (H.E stain)

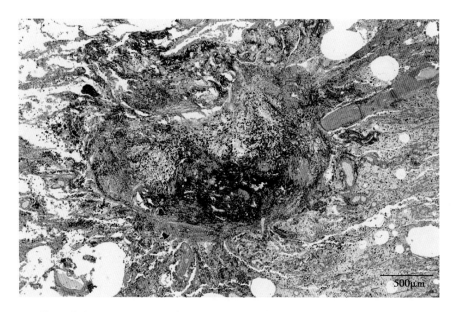

图 90　煤矽结节:结节内大量胶原纤维分布,可见煤尘沉积在胶原纤维之间。纤维性"伪足"向周边伸延,周围肺泡腔内浆液渗出。(掘进、采煤工作 26 年)(H.E 染色)

Fig.90　Coal silicotic nodule: A large amount of collagen fibers, mixing with coal dust, grow in the nodule. The pseudopodia-shaped collagen fibers protrude from the lesion and extend toward the pulmonary tissue. The alveolar space surrounding the lesion is filled with serous exudation. (From the patient, working in the coal tunneling and mining for 26 years) (H.E stain)

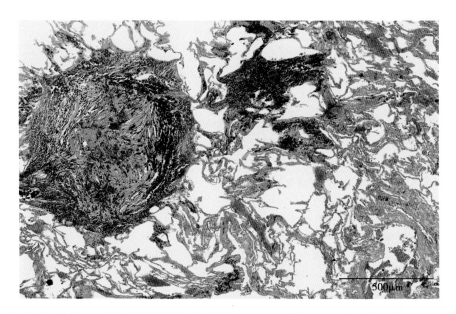

图 91　煤矽结节:结节内大量胶原纤维呈"洋葱皮样"分布,可见煤尘沉积在结节外侧带呈"套袖样"结构。结节临近有一煤尘纤维灶。(掘进工作 20 年)(H.E 染色)

Fig.91　Coal silicotic nodule: Heavily deposited collagen in the nodule is shown as the pink laminated appearance, and the aggregated coal dust border the periphery of the lesion, looking like a "cuff-cover". In adjacent to the lesion, a cellular coal dust fibrous nodule is found. (From the patient, working in coal tunneling for 20 years) (H.E stain)

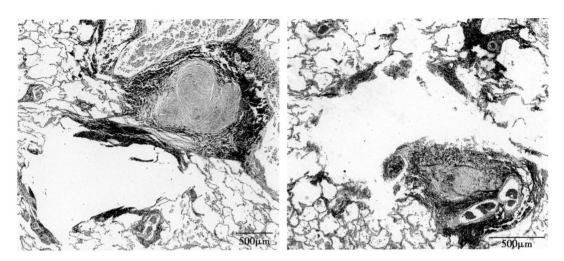

图92 煤矽结节:结节内胶原纤维呈玻璃样变性,尘细胞沉积在结节内或外侧带呈"袖套样"环绕,结节向呼吸性细支气管腔内突入,伴呼吸性细支气管扩张。(掘进工作20年)(H.E染色)

Fig.92 Coal silicotic nodule: The collagen in the nodule develops to be hyaline change and coal dust-laden macrophages distribute in the lesion or are aggregated surrounding the hyaline collagen, looking like a "cuff-cover". The nodule also penetrates into an enlarged respiratory bronchiole lumen. (From the patient, performing on the coal tunneling for 20 years) (H.E stain)

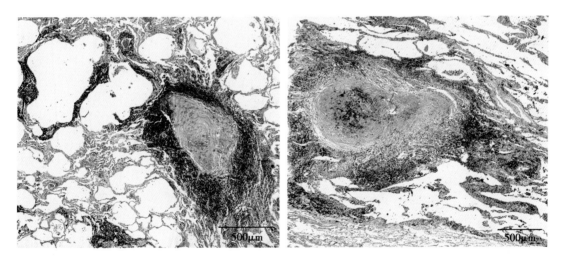

图93 煤矽结节:结节内胶原纤维呈"洋葱皮"样分布。可见煤尘细胞沉积在结节外侧带呈"套袖样"环绕,伴肺气肿形成。(左图,掘进工作20年;右图,井下凿岩工作20年)(H.E染色)

Fig.93 Coal silicotic nodule: In the nodule, the collagen arranged in laminated way is surrounded by coal dust-laden macrophages, looking like a "cuff-cover". Meanwhile, the lung has emphysema change.〔From the patients, working in coal tunneling for 20 years (left) and in the coal rock drilling work for 20 years (right)〕(H.E stain)

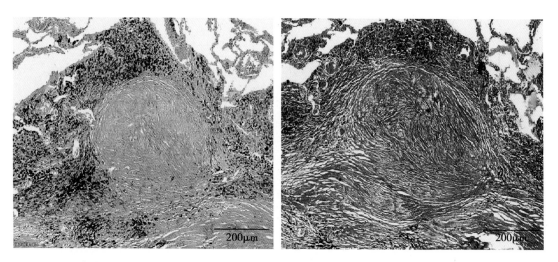

图 94　煤矽结节：左图，纤维化的结节玻璃样变性，可见条索状分布及融合的胶原纤维位于结节中央，煤尘沉积在结节外侧带呈"套袖样"环绕(H.E 染色)。右图，结节内蓝色条索状结构为胶原纤维。(Masson 染色) (井下凿岩工作 20 年)

Fig.94　Coal silicotic nodule: (Left) In the nodule, the collagen arranged in laminated way is surrounded by the aggregated coal dust cells, looking like a "cuff-cover". (H.E stain) (Right) The collagen fibers in the nodule are stained with blue color. (Masson stain) (From the patient, working in coal rock drilling for 20 years)

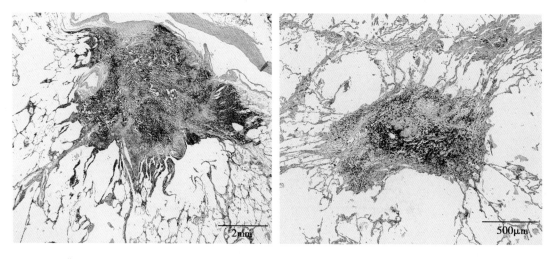

图 95　不典型煤矽结节：肺内较大的不规则结节状病灶，结节内大量胶原纤维(≥结节面积 50%)和较多煤尘沉积，纤维状伪足向四周肺组织中伸延，伴灶周肺气肿形成。(井下采煤工作 4 年，井上其他混合工作 20 年)(H.E 染色)

Fig.95　Atypical coal silicotic nodule: The lung shows a mildly larger, irregular nodular lesion, composing of coal dust-laden macrophages and abundant collagen fibers (the collagen area is over 50% of whole lesion). The pseudopodia-shaped fibrous tissue protrudes from the lesion and extends toward the surrounding tissue. It is accompanied with emphysema formation. (From the patient, working in coal mining for 4 years and ground service for 20 years) (H.E stain)

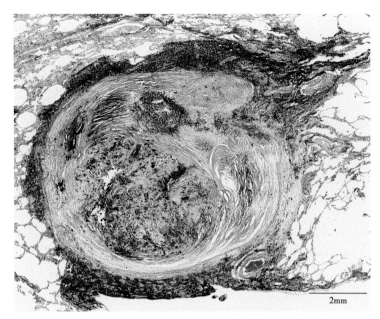

2mm

图 96 融合型煤矽结节：由一个较大和多个较小的结节融合在一起构成。（采煤工作 29 年）（H.E 染色）

Fig.96 Confluent coal silicotic nodules: The massive coal silicotic nodule is created by one larger coal silicotic nodule and several small ones. (From the patient, working in coal mining working for 29 years) (H.E stain)

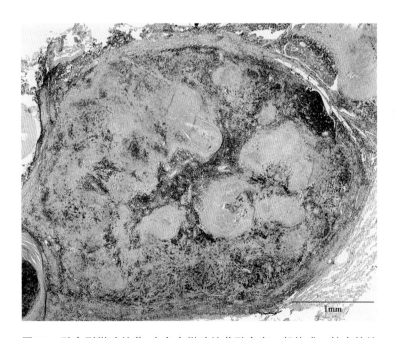

1mm

图 97 融合型煤矽结节：由多个煤矽结节融合在一起构成一较大的结节。（采煤工作 29 年）（H.E 染色）

Fig.97 Confluent coal silicotic nodules: Several coal silicotic nodules merge to a larger coal silicotic nodule. (From the patient, working in coal mining working for 29 years) (H.E stain)

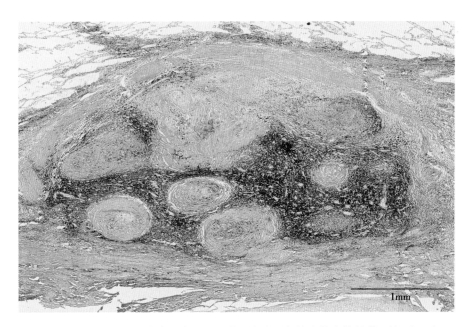

图 98　融合型煤矽结节：肺内多个煤矽结节融合在一起构成较大的结节。(掘进工作 20 年)(H.E 染色)

Fig.98　Confluent coal silicotic nodules: A bigger coal silicotic nodule is the result of many coal silicotic nodules fusion. (From the patient, working in coal tunneling for 20 years) (H.E stain)

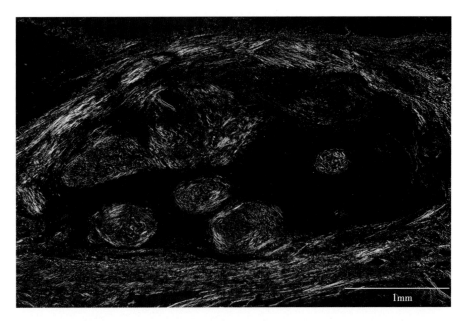

图 99　融合型煤矽结节(与图 98 同一视野)：黄色为分布的Ⅰ型胶原，绿色为分布的Ⅲ型胶原。(天狼猩红染色，偏振光观察)

Fig.99　Confluent coal silicotic nodules (same microscopic field as Fig. 98): Collagen type I is stained with orange color, and collagen type III shows green color. (Sirius red stain, polarization light microscope with dark field)

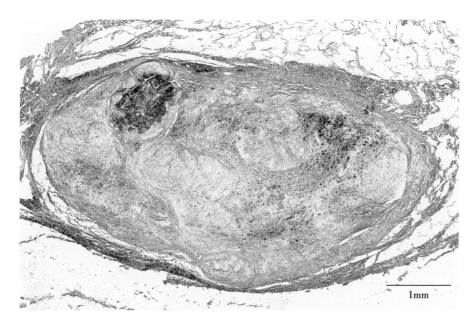

图 100　融合型煤矽结节：结节内大量胶原沉积伴玻璃样变性，可见较多煤尘沉积在结节内和结节外侧。（掘进工作 20 年）（H.E 染色）

Fig.100　Confluent coal silicotic nodule: Abundant collagen fibers with hyaline change could be seen in the nodules. Coal dust deposits within or around the lesion. (From the patient, performing on coal tunneling for 20 years) (H.E stain)

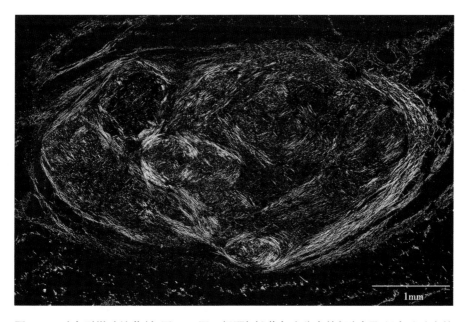

图 101　融合型煤矽结节（与图 100 同一视野）：橙黄色为分布的 I 型胶原，绿色为分布的 Ⅲ 型胶原。（天狼猩红染色，偏振光观察）

Fig.101　Confluent coal silicotic nodule (same microscopic field as Fig.100): Collagen type I is stained with orange color, while collagen type Ⅲ shows green color. (Sirius red stain, polarization light microscope with dark field)

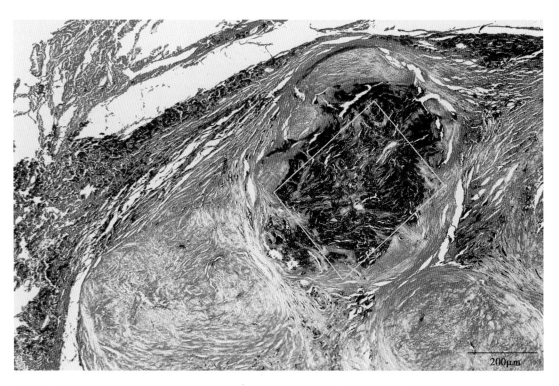

图 102　肺内融合型煤矽结节。(掘进工作 20 年)(天狼星红染色,偏振光观察,明场)
Fig.102　Confluent coal silicotic nodules. (Sirius red stain, polarization light microscope with light field) (From the patient, working in coal tunneling for 20 years)

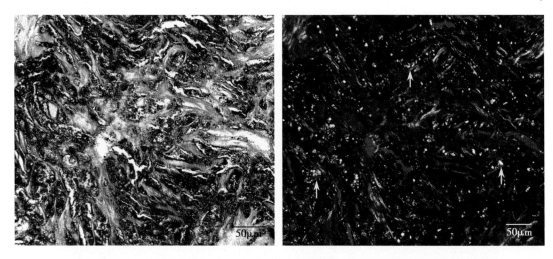

图 103　肺内融合型煤矽结节(图 102 局部放大):左图(天狼星红染色,偏振光观察,明场),右图(天狼星红染色,偏振光观察,暗场)可见在增生的胶原纤维(橙色为Ⅰ型胶原,绿色为Ⅲ型胶原)间有较多折光性强的矽(煤)尘颗粒(箭头所指)。
Fig.103　Confluent coal silicotic nodules (regional amplification of Fig 102): Note dense collagen, presenting at the confluent coal silicotic nodules of both left photography (sirius red stain staining, polarized light microscopy) and right one (sirius red stain, polarized dark microscopy), where collagen type I is highlighted as orange, collagen type Ⅲ is green and silica (coal) particles shows strong power of refraction (arrows).

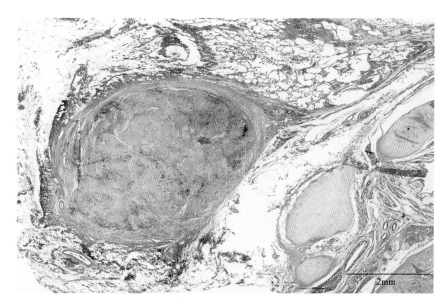

图 104 矽结节：肺内支气管旁矽结节内大量胶原沉积并发生玻璃样变性，仅见较少量煤尘沉积在结节内和外围。（井下测量工作 15 年）（H.E 染色）

Fig.104 Silicotic nodule: A large amount of collagen fibers of nodule undergo hyaline change. In contrary to the silicotic (coal) nodules, coal dust is hardly to be seen in the silicotic nodules. This figure provides the evidence that less amount of coal dust scatters within or around the nodule. (From the patient, performing on underground survey for 15 years) (H.E stain)

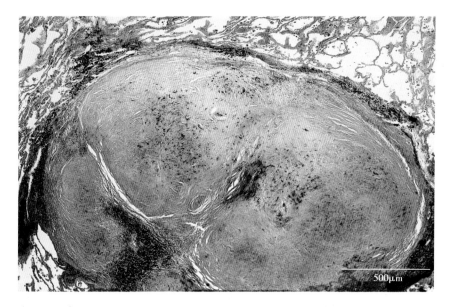

图 105 融合型矽结节：由三个结节融合组成。结节内大量胶原沉积并发生玻璃样变性，可见部分煤尘沉积在结节内和结节外侧。（井下测量工作 15 年）（HE 染色）

Fig.105 Confluent silicotic nodules: The confluent silicotic nodule is developed by three smaller nodules coalescence, showing a large amount of collagen fibers with hyaline change and coal dust aggregation within or around the lesion. (From the patient, performing on underground survey for 15 years) (H.E stain)

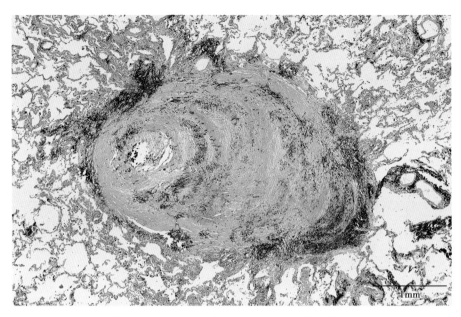

图 106　矽结节:结节内玻璃样变性的胶原纤维与煤尘交替层状分布,并可见一个管壁增厚的小血管。(采煤、掘进、运输工作 31 年)(H.E 染色)

Fig.106　Silicotic nodule: It alternates the layer of hyaline collagen fibers and deposited coal dusts in the silicotic nodule. Note a small blood vessel with thicken wall in the nodule. (From the patient, serving the mine for 31 years to perform coal mining, tunneling and transportation works) (H.E stain)

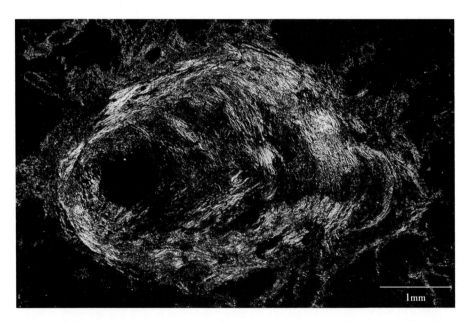

图 107　矽结节(与图 106 同一视野):橙黄色为分布的Ⅰ型胶原,绿色为分布的Ⅲ型胶原。(天狼猩红染色,偏振光观察)

Fig.107　Silicotic nodule (same microscopic field as Fig. 102): Collagen type I is stained with orange color, while collagen type III shows green color. (Sirius red stain, polarization light macroscope with dark field)

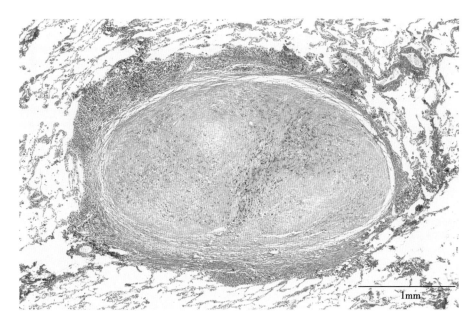

图 108 矽结节:结节内大量胶原沉积并发生玻璃样变性,可见少量煤尘沉积在结节内和结节外侧。(井下测量工作 15 年)(H.E 染色)

Fig.108 Silicotic nodule: Abundant collagen fibers with hyaline change are visible in the nodules. A small amount of coal dust deposits within or around the lesion. (From the patient, performing on underground survey for 15 years) (H.E stain)

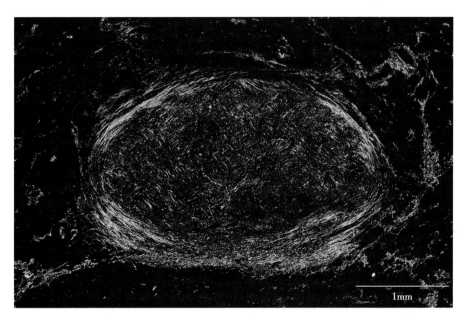

图 109 矽结节(与图 108 同一视野):橙黄色为分布的I型胶原,绿色为分布的Ⅲ型胶原。(天狼猩红染色,偏振光观察)

Fig.109 Silicotic nodule (same microscopic field as Fig.106): Collagen type I is stained with orange color, and collagen type III shows green color. (Sirius red stain, polarization light microscope with dark field)

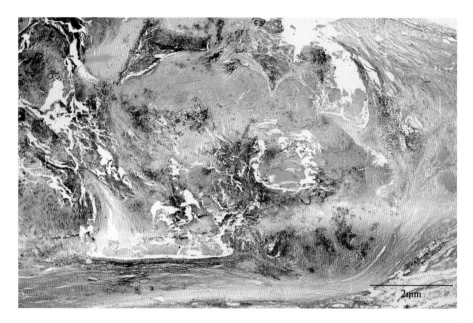

图110 进行性块状纤维化:团块由大量弥漫增生的胶原纤维与沉积在其间的煤尘构成。胶原纤维玻璃样变性。(岩凿工作 32 年)(H.E 染色)

Fig.110 Progressive massive fibrosis: Diffuse fibrous proliferation with hyaline change and deposits of coal dust form an extensive mass. (From the patient, working in rock drilling for 32 years) (H.E stain)

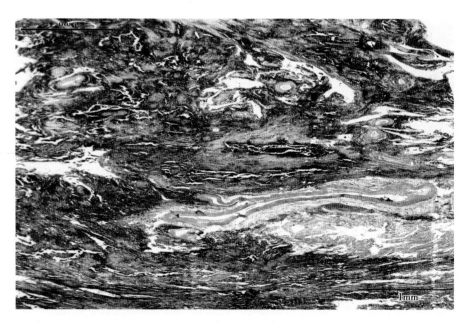

图 111 进行性块状纤维化:大量煤尘沉积,伴纤维组织弥漫增生形成团块状结构。(掘进工作 20 年)(H.E 染色)

Fig.111 Progressive massive fibrosis: The lesion is formed by abundant coal dust deposits with diffuse fibrous proliferation. (From the patient, working in coal tunneling for 20 years) (H.E stain)

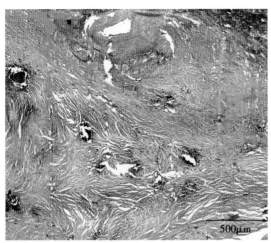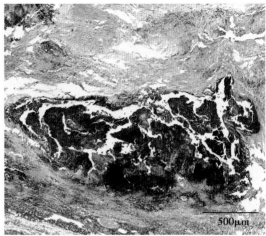

图112 进行性块状纤维化：团块内粗大的胶原纤维弥漫分布，条索状交错编织状走行，部分纤维玻璃样变，其中煤尘在胶原纤维间沉积。右图显示大量煤尘局灶性聚集形成较大的煤尘池。（左图采煤工作22年，右图掘进工作20年）（H.E染色）

Fig.112 Progressive massive fibrous lesion: Characteristic storiform pattern of collagen with hyaline change intersperses with scattered coal dust deposits. Note a larger "coal dust pool" of abundant coal dust deposition in the right photography.〔From the patients, working in coal mining for 22 years (left) and in coal tunneling for 20 years (right)〕(H.E stain)

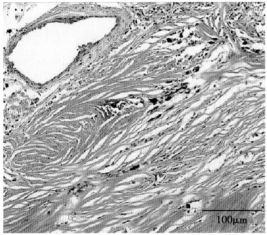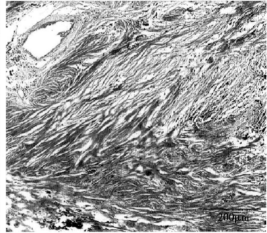

图113 进行性块状纤维化：左图，团块内粗大的胶原纤维弥漫分布，条索状交错编织状走行，部分纤维玻璃样变，可见煤尘在胶原纤维间沉积（H.E染色）；右图，胶原纤维呈蓝色（采煤工作21年）（Massson染色）

Fig. 113 Progressive massive fibrous lesion: (Left) H.E section of massive fibrous lesion, illustrates the storiform pattern of collagen with hyaline change interspersed with scattered coal dust deposits in the left photography. (Right) Masson stain to accentuate the collagen with blue color in the right one. (From the patients, working in coal mining for 21 years)

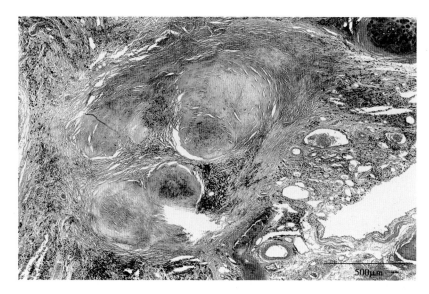

图 114　融合型块状纤维化：纤维性团块由融合性矽结节与增生的纤维组织构成。结节发生玻璃样变性，增生的胶原呈交错编织状走行于结节间与结节外围，其间较多煤尘沉积在结节周围与胶原纤维间。（回采、掘进工作 17 年）（H.E 染色）

Fig.114　Confluent massive fibrous lesion: The fibrous lesion contains confluent silica nodules with hyaline change and proliferated fibrous tissues in a storiform pattern, which distributes inside and outside the lesion. Minimal coal dust deposits either around the silica nodules or between the collagen. (From the patient, working in coal mining and tunneling for 17 years) (H.E stain)

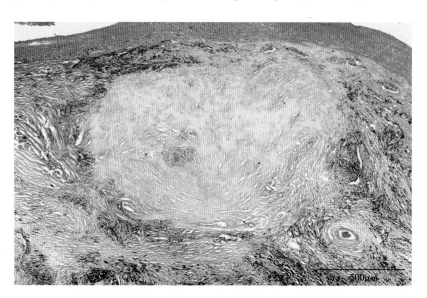

图 115　融合型块状纤维化：团块由矽结节与增生的纤维组织融合在一起构成。煤尘细胞在结节周围与胶原纤维间沉积。（与图 114 同一病例）（H.E 染色）

Fig.115　Confluent massive fibrous lesion: The lesion is composed of the fusion of silicotic nodules and proliferated fibrous tissue. Coal dust-laden macrophages deposit around the silica nodules and between collagen fibers. (Sample is same as Fig. 114) (H.E stain)

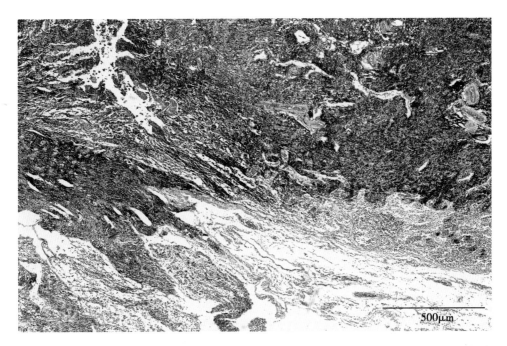

图116　弥漫性尘性间质纤维化：肺间质大量煤尘沉积伴纤维组织增生，并形成"伪足"向邻近肺组织伸延，伴小血管增生充血。（采煤工作24年）（H.E染色）

Fig.116　Diffuse coal interstitial fibrosis: Histologic appearance of pulmonary interstitial tissue with abundant coal dust deposits, proliferated fibrous tissue and congested small blood vessels, extending to the adjacent tissues in a spike pattern. (H.E stain) (From the patient, working in coal mining for 24 years)

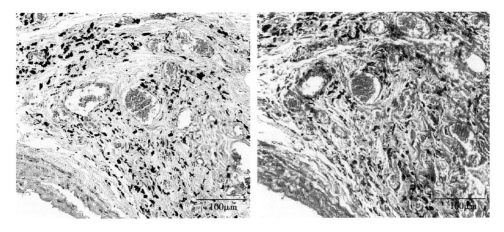

图117　弥漫性尘性间质纤维化：左图（HE染色），肺间质胶原纤维增生弥漫分布。其间可见小血管的增生、充血，煤尘沉积在胶原纤维间。右图（Masson染色），蓝色显示增生的胶原纤维。（采煤工作22年）

Fig.117　Diffuse coal interstitial fibrosis: (Left) H.E section of lung shows the interstitial fibrous hyperplasia in a diffusely scattered patten, alternated proliferated and congested small blood vessels as well as moderate amount of coal dust. (Right) Masson stain is to highlight collagen fibers as blue color. (From the patient, working in coal mining for 22 years)

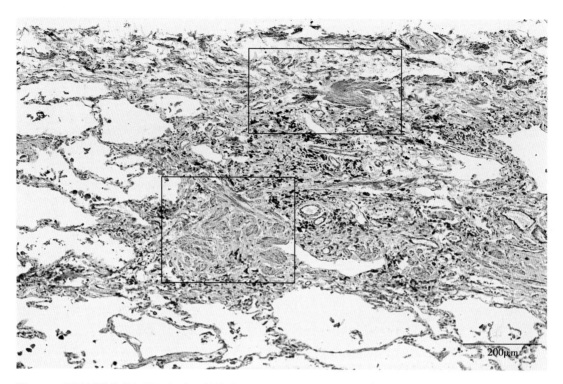

图 118　间质纤维化伴平滑肌细胞局灶性增生：在弥漫性增生的纤维组织中可见 α- 平滑肌肌动蛋白阳性表达的细胞团块状增生。（井下测量工作 15 年）（α- 平滑肌肌动蛋白免疫组化染色）

Fig.118　Interstitial fibrosis with local proliferated smooth muscle cells: Massive pattern of cells with positive expression of α-smooth muscle actin (α-SMA) is visible in the diffuse proliferated fibrous tissue. (From the patient, working in underground survey for 15 years) (α-SMA immunohistochemical stain)

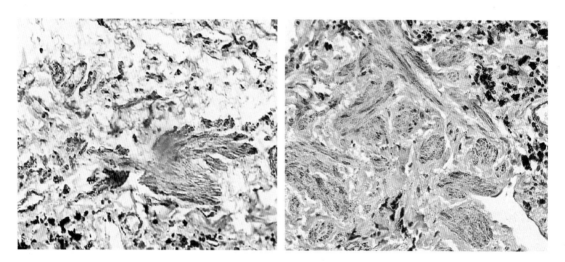

图 119　间质纤维化伴平滑肌细胞局灶性增生（图 118 局部放大）：棕黄色为 α- 平滑肌肌动蛋白阳性标记的增生的平滑肌细胞。

Fig.119　Interstitial fibrosis with local proliferated smooth muscle cells (regional amplification of Fig.116): The proliferated smooth muscle cells are denoted by brown-yellow color, which indicates positive expression of α-smooth muscle actin.

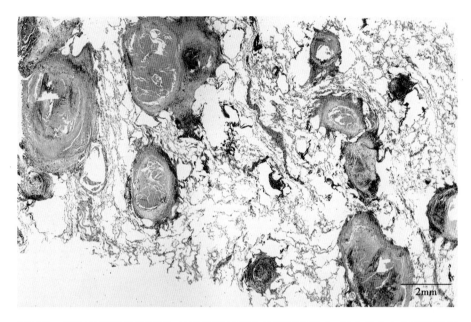

图 120　煤工尘肺伴结核病变：结核结节与煤矽结节病变融合，形成多个大小不等的煤矽结核结节分布在肺内。（掘进、岩凿工作 20 年）（H.E 染色）
Fig.120　Coal workers' pneumoconiosis with tuberculosis: Tubercles are able to fuse with coal silicotic nodules, forming various-sized silicotic tuberculous nodules in lung. (From the patient, working in coal tunneling and rock drilling for 20 years) (H.E stain)

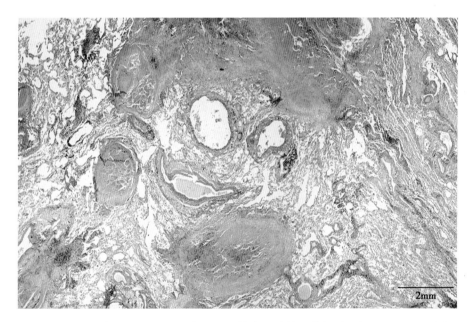

图 121　煤工尘肺伴结核病变：多个大小不等煤矽结核结节与煤尘纤维灶分布在肺内，伴局部团块状间质纤维化形成。（与图 120 同一病例）（H.E 染色）
Fig.121　Coal workers' pneumoconiosis with tuberculosis: Coal silicotic tuberculous nodules in different size, with mosaiced coal fibrous foci, are visible in lung. Note a focal massive interstitial fibrosis. (Sample is same as Fig.120) (H.E stain)

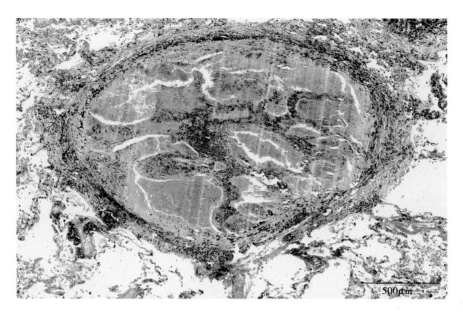

图 122 肺内早期煤矽结核结节：结节中央部为干酪样坏死物充填在肺泡腔内，煤尘沉积在肺泡壁。结节外侧为增生的纤维组织与煤尘构成的"套袖样"结构。（掘进、井下运输工作 22 年）（H.E 染色）

Fig.122 Early stage of coal silicotic tuberculous nodule: There is central caseous necrosis filled in alveolar space and coal dust deposited in alveolar septum, with a surrounding rim of proliferated collagen fibers and coal dust deposits, forming a "cuff-cover" appearance. (From the patient, working in coal tunneling and transportation for 22 years) (H.E stain)

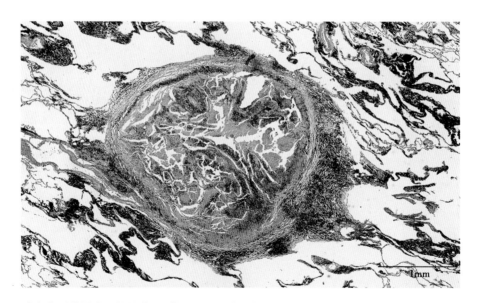

图 123 肺内典型的煤矽结核结节：结节中央为干酪样坏死和煤尘的混合，外周为胶原纤维及煤尘沉积构成"套袖样"结构，周围肺组织尘性间质纤维化和肺气肿形成。（井下采煤 8 年，井上其他混合工作 8 年）（H.E 染色）

Fig.123 Classic coal silicotic tuberculous nodule: Caseous necrosis and coal dust are surrounded by the mixture of collagen fibers and coal dust, forming a "cuff-cover" appearance. Note interstitial coal fibrosis and emphysema in adjacent tissue. (From the patient, performing coal mining and ground service for 8 years respectively) (H.E stain)

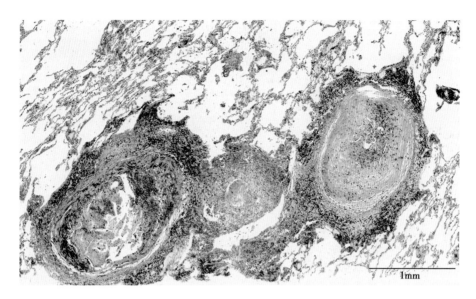

图 124　肺内煤矽结核结节：两侧两个典型煤矽结核结节。结节中心为结核性干酪样坏死，外周为呈层状分布增生的胶原纤维以及煤尘沉积形成的"套袖样"结构。中央结节为不典型煤矽结核结节。（掘进、岩凿工作 20 年）（H.E 染色）

Fig.124　Coal silicotic tuberculous nodules: Microscopic view of two classic coal silicotic tuberculous nodules and one atypical nodule in between. Located at the center of classic nodules are extensive areas of caseous necrosis, and the outer layer is laminated proliferated collagen fibers combined with coal dust, forming a "cuff-cover" appearance. (From the patient, working in coal tunneling and rock drilling for 20 years) (H.E stain)

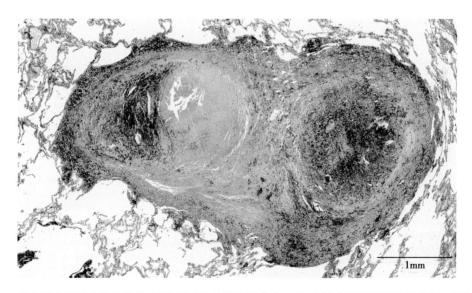

图 125　肺内融合型煤矽结核结节：两个煤矽结核结节融合在一起，由增生的胶原纤维及煤尘沉积构成，其中左侧结节中心为结核性干酪样坏死。（与图 124 同一病例）（H.E 染色）

Fig.125　Confluent coal silicotic tuberculous nodules: Photography illustrating coal silicotic tuberculous nodule created by the fusion of two small ones, containing proliferated collagen fibers and deposited coal dust. The left is marked by the central caseous necrosis. (Sample is same as Fig.124) (H.E stain)

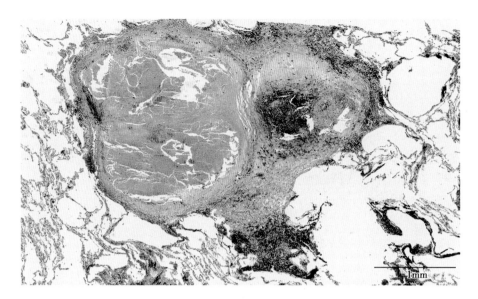

图 126　肺内融合型煤矽结核结节：两个煤矽结核结节融合在一起，由增生的胶原纤维以及煤尘沉积构成，其中左侧结节中心为较大面积的结核性干酪样坏死。(掘进、岩凿工作 20 年)(H.E 染色)

Fig.126　Confluent coal silicotic tuberculous nodules: Two coal silicotic tuberculous nodules are growing into a coalescence lesion, containing abundant collagen fibers and coal dust. Note an extensive area of caseous necrosis in the middle of the left one. (From the patient, working in coal tunneling and rock drilling for 20 years) (H.E stain)

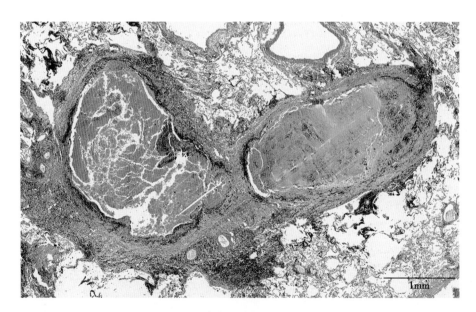

图 127　肺内融合型煤矽结核结节：两个煤矽结核结节融合，由增生的胶原纤维及煤尘沉积构成，结节中心为较大面积的结核性干酪样坏死。(掘进、井下运输工作 22 年)(H.E 染色)

Fig.127　Confluent coal silicotic tuberculous nodules: Photography showing coalescence of two coal silicotic tuberculous nodules with central extensive caseous necrosis and surrounding dense collagen and deposited coal dust. (From the patient, working in coal tunneling and underground transportation for 22 years) (H.E stain)

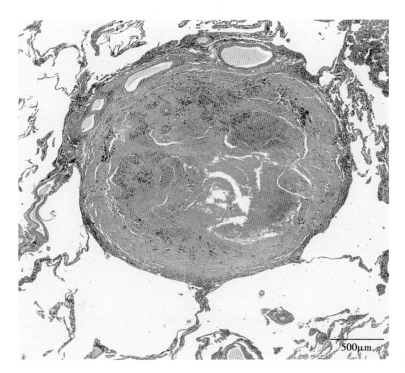

图 128　煤工尘肺矽结核结节：结节外侧为层状增生的胶原纤维和少量煤尘沉积混合构成，中心区域可见较大面积的干酪样坏死。（掘进工作 17 年）（H.E 染色）

Fig.128　Silicotic tuberculous nodules of coal works' pneumoconiosis: A well demarcated nodule is composed of central massive caseous necrosis and the surrounding mixture of proliferated collagen fibers and minimal coal dust. (From the patient, working in coal tunneling for 17 years) (H.E stain)

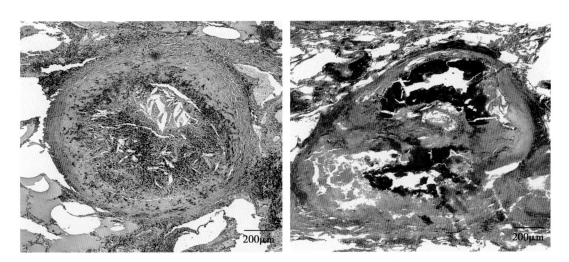

图 129　煤工尘肺矽结核结节：左图显示结节由层状增生的胶原纤维和煤尘沉积混合构成，中心区域可见干酪样坏死与胆固醇结晶的析出。右图显示结节中央大面积干酪样坏死伴钙化形成。（岩凿工作 7 年）（H.E 染色）

Fig.129　Silicotic tuberculous nodules of coal works' pneumoconiosis: Photographys show central caseous necrosis, combined with cholesterol crystals (left) or calcification response (right), is surrounded by the mixture of proliferated collagen fibers and coal dust. (From the patient, working in rock drilling for 7 years) (H.E stain)

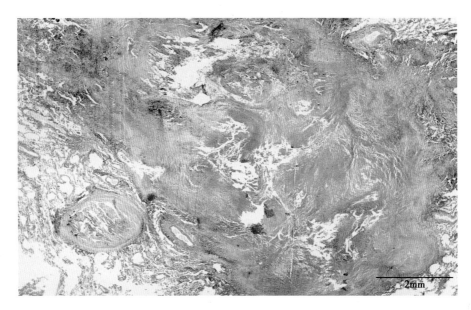

图 130　结节融合型块状纤维化：由多个矽结核结节融合形成纤维化团块病灶。(掘进、岩凿工作 20 年)(H.E 染色)

Fig.130　Nodular confluent massive fibrosis: A massive fibrous lesion is created by coalescence of multiple silicotic tuberculous nodules. (From the patient, working in coal tunneling and rock drilling for 20 years) (H.E stain)

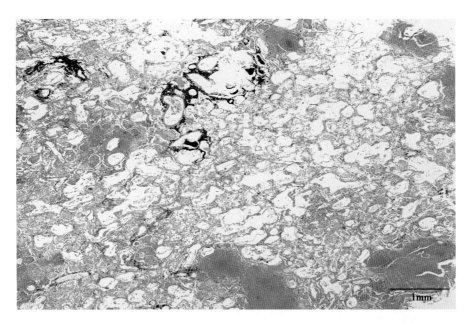

图 131　煤工尘肺伴播散性粟粒性肺结核：肺内煤尘斑 - 气肿病变,伴多个干酪样坏死实变病灶。(掘进、井下运输工作 22 年)(H.E 染色)

Fig.131　Disseminated miliary tuberculosis of coal workers' pneumoconiosis: In the background of coalworkers' pneumoconiosis (coal maculae and emphysemas), multiple consolidated tubercles with caseous necrosis are visible. (From the patient, working in coal tunneling and underground transportion for 22 years) (H.E stain)

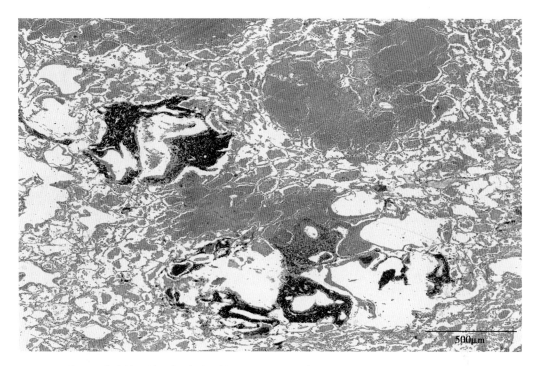

图 132 煤工尘肺伴播散性粟粒性肺结核：煤斑（灶）- 肺气肿病变，伴干酪样坏死实变病灶形成。病灶周围肺泡腔内充满大量干酪样坏死物和炎性渗出物。（井下机电维修工作 20 年）（H.E 染色）

Fig.132 Disseminated miliary tuberculosis of coal workers' pneumoconiosis: Microscopic view illustration of coal dust dots and foci surrounded by emphysemas, accompanied by consolidated caseous necrosis. Note extensive caseous necrosis and inflammatory exudates filled in the surrounding airspace. (From the patient, working in underground maintenance of equipment and electricity for 20 years) (H.E stain)

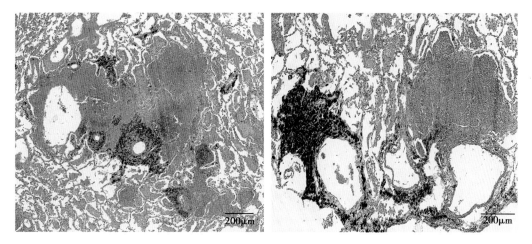

图 133 煤工尘肺伴播散性粟粒性肺结核：肺内煤尘细胞灶，伴干酪样坏死实变病灶形成。（与图 132 同一病例）（H.E 染色）

Fig.133 Disseminated miliary tuberculosis of coalworkers' pneumoconiosis: Coal dust cell foci and consolidated caseous necrosis lesions are visible in lung. (Sample is same as Fig.132) (H.E stain)

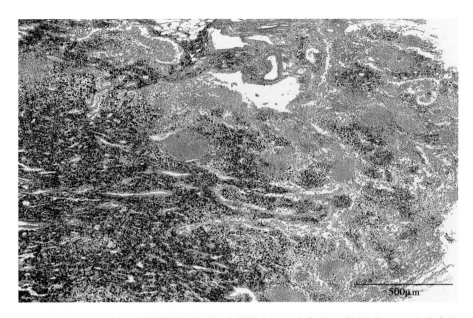

图 134　煤工尘肺伴播散性粟粒性肺结核:大量煤尘沉积肺内伴间质纤维化,可见多个类圆形干酪样坏死病灶和结核性肉芽肿病变分布在肺内。(井下机电维修工作 20 年)(H.E 染色)

Fig.134　Disseminated miliary tuberculosis of coalworkers' pneumoconiosis: Showing severe coal dust deposition in the fibrous interstitial tissue, scattered quasi-circular caseous necrosis lesions and tuberculous granulomas. (From the patient, working in underground maintenance of equipment and electricity for 20 years) (H.E stain)

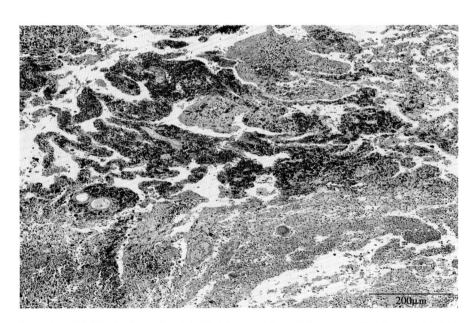

图 135　尘性结核性结节:肺内大量煤尘沉积,煤尘灶形成,伴间质纤维化,肺内可见结核性肉芽肿病变。(与图 134 同一病例)(H.E 染色)

Fig.135　Coal dust tuberculous nodules: Changes of coalworkers' pneumoconiosis (coal dust deposits and coal dust-laden macrophages foci), are associated with tuberculosis granulomas (nodular granulomas) and interstitial fibrosis. (Sample is same as Fig.134.) (H.E stain)

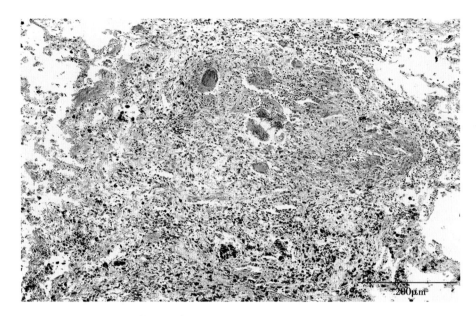

图 136　尘性结核性肉芽肿(结节):由增生的上皮样细胞、郎罕氏多核巨细胞及其煤尘混杂在一起构成。(井下机电维修工作 20 年)(H.E 染色)

Fig.136　Coal dust tuberculous granuloma (nodule): The granulomas are characterized by proliferated epithelioid cells, Langhans giant cells and deposited coal dusts. (From the patient, working in underground maintenance of equipment and electricity for 20 years) (H.E stain)

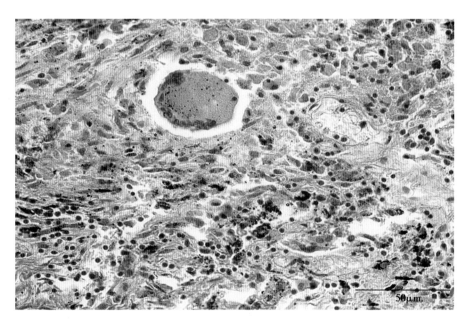

图 137　尘性结核性肉芽肿(结节):郎罕氏多核巨细胞胞浆内可见煤尘颗粒。(与图 136 同一病例)(H.E 染色)

Fig.137　Coal dust tuberculous granuloma (nodule): Coal dust particles are present in cytoplasm of Langhans giant cells. (Sample is same as Fig.136) (H.E stain)

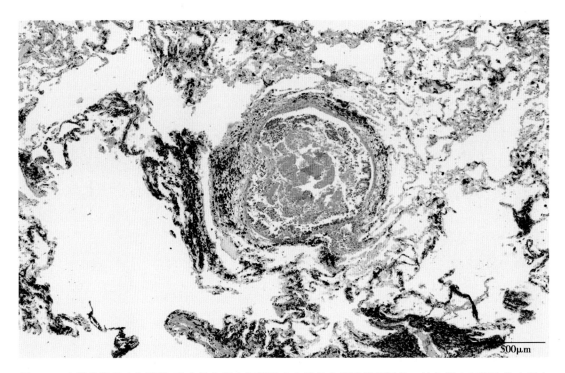

图 138　尘性结核性支气管炎:肺内终末细支气管腔内充填较多干酪样坏死物。较多煤尘沉积在终末细支气管壁外侧及呼吸性细支气管,伴呼吸性细支气管扩张。(掘进工作 17 年)(H.E 染色)
Fig.138　Coal dust tuberculous bronchiolitis: Terminal bronchiole lumen is filled with caseous necrosis, with coal dust deposition in the wall. Note the dilated respiratory bronchioles are also deposited by coal dust. (From the patient, working in coal tunneling for 17 years) (H.E staining)

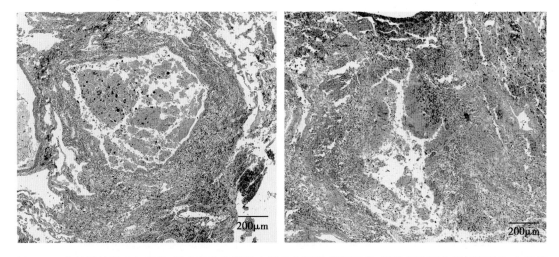

图 139　尘性结核性支气管炎:肺内细支气管腔充填较多干酪样坏死物,管壁郎格罕多核巨细胞和大量炎细胞浸润,其间夹杂着煤尘细胞。(掘进、井下运输工作 22 年)(H.E 染色)
Fig.139　Coal dust tuberculous bronchiolitis: Microscopic illustration of caseous necrosis filled in bronchioles lumen, with infiltrate of Langhans giant cells, inflammatory cells and coal dust cells in bronchioles wall. (From the patient, working in coal tunneling and underground transportation for 22 years) (H.E stain)

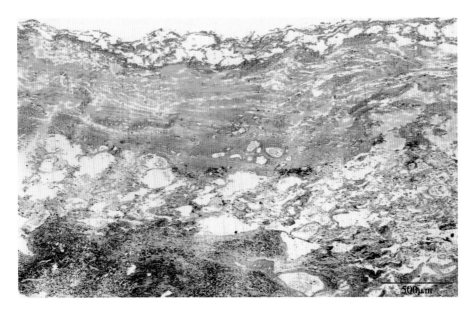

图 140　煤工尘肺伴结核性胸膜炎：煤尘沉积的肺组织表面覆盖大量纤维素样渗出物，胸膜增厚。（与图 139 同一病例）（H.E 染色）

Fig.140　Tuberculous pleuritis of coal workers' pneumoconiosis: Deposits of fibrin on the pleura. Note coal dust deposits under the pleura. (Sample is same as Fig.139) (H.E stain)

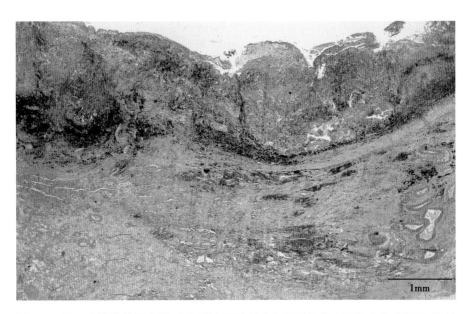

图 141　煤工尘肺结核性空洞：空洞壁内侧为煤尘与干酪样坏死物混杂构成坏死层，其外侧为纤维组织构成的纤维层，与间质纤维化的肺组织相移行，相邻肺组织弥漫变实，伴发其它细菌感染。（与图 140 同一病例）（H.E 染色）

Fig. 141　Tuberculous cavity of coal workers' pneumoconiosis: Microscopic view of tuberculous cavity wall, demonstrating the inner necrotic layer, composed of caseous necrosis and coal dust deposits, and outer fibrous layer of a dense collagen, jointing with disseminated consolidated pulmonary tissue with other bacterial infection. (Sample is same as Fig.140) (H.E stain)

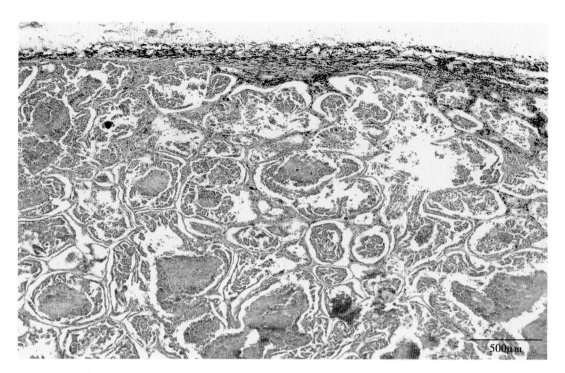

图 142 煤工尘肺伴发肺腺癌:较多煤尘沉积在胸膜,胸膜增厚。 胸膜直下为癌组织,呈腺泡样结构。部分腺泡样癌巢中心组织发生坏死。(掘进、采煤工作 25 年)(H.E 染色)

Fig.142 Coal workers' pneumoconiosis with pulmonary adenocarcinoma: The thickening pleura is response to coal dust deposits. Subpleural pulmonary tissue is replaced by acinar carcinoma nests, some of which is marked by a central zone of necrosis. (From the patient, working in coal tunneling and mining for 25 years) (H.E stain)

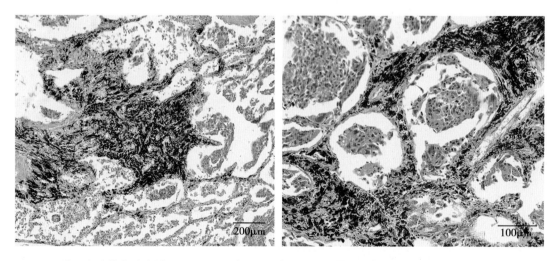

图 143 煤工尘肺伴发腺癌(与图 142 同一病例):细胞纤维性结节周围为腺癌组织(左图)。煤尘沉积在肺泡壁与间质中,肺泡腔内充填癌组织(右图)。(H.E 染色)

Fig.143 Coal workers' pneumoconiosis with pulmonary adenocarcinoma: Left photography evidence of cellular fibrotic nodules surrounded by adenocarcinoma tissue. Right photography showing adenocarcinoma filled in alveolar space, with coal dust deposition in alveolar wall and interstitial tissue. (Sample is same as Fig.142) (H.E stain)

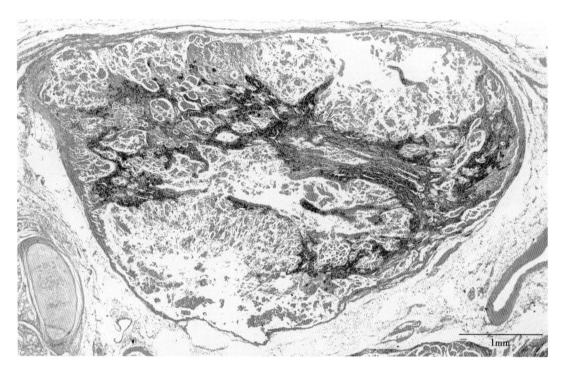

图 144　煤工尘肺伴淋巴结转移腺癌：支气管旁淋巴结内煤尘沉积伴间质纤维化。腺癌组织转移到淋巴结伴大量组织坏死，破坏淋巴结原有结构。（与图 142 同一病例）（H.E 染色）

Fig.144　Coal workers' pneumoconiosis with lymph node adenocarcinoma metastasis: The peribronchial lymph node with coal dust deposition and interstitial fibrosis is destroyed by adenocarcinomae, producing extensive necrotic tissue. (Sample is same as Fig.142) (H.E stain)

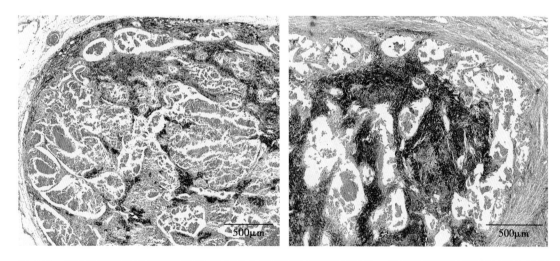

图 145　煤工尘肺伴淋巴结转移腺癌：淋巴结内煤尘沉积伴间质纤维化。腺癌组织转移到淋巴结伴组织坏死，破坏淋巴结原有结构。（与图 144 同一病例）（H.E 染色）

Fig.145　Coal workers' pneumoconiosis with lymph node adenocarcinoma metastasis: Schematic illustration of coal dust deposition and interstitial fibrosis in lymph nodes, with normal tissue destruction by adenocarcinoma cells, showing tissue necrosis. (Sample is same as Fig.144) (H.E stain)

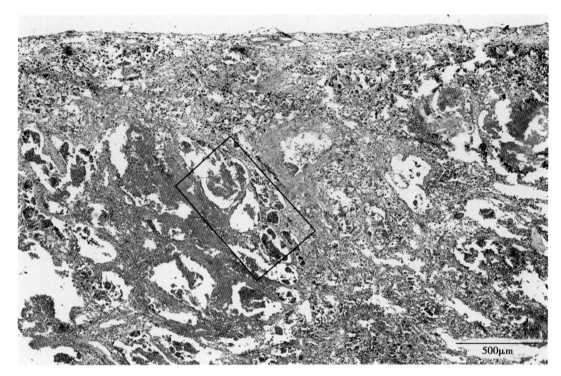

图 146 煤工尘肺伴发肺腺癌：一些煤尘沉积在胸膜及胸膜下方,胸膜增厚。胸膜直下为癌组织,呈腺泡样结构。部分腺泡样癌巢中心组织发生坏死,伴间质纤维组织增生。(掘进工作 17 年)(H.E 染色)

Fig.146 Coal workers' pneumoconiosis with pulmonary adenocarcinoma: The thickening pleura is accumulated with coal dust deposits. Subpleural pulmonary tissue is replaced by coal dust deposits, proliferated collagen fibers and adenocarcinoma with gland formation that has occasional central necrotic actions. (From the patient, working in coal tunneling for 17 years) (H.E stain)

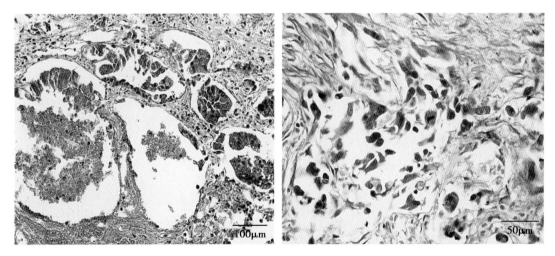

图 147 煤工尘肺伴发肺腺癌：左图为上图局部放大。右图为异性的肿瘤细胞。(H.E 染色)

Fig.147 Coal workers' pneumoconiosis with pulmonary adenocarcinoma: (Left) Regional amplification of Fig. 146. (Right) Malignant tumor cells with obvious atypia. (H.E stain)

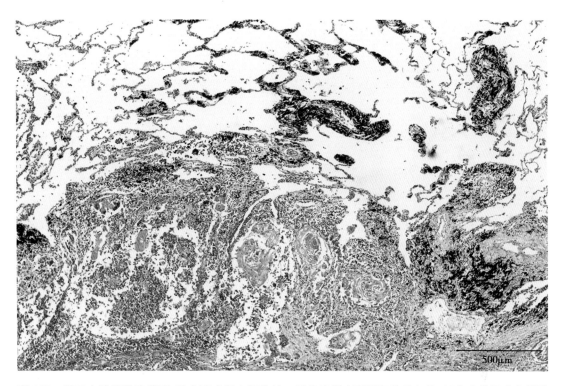

图 148 煤工尘肺伴发腺鳞癌：肺内形成煤尘细胞灶。部分癌巢中可见细胞的角化，部分癌巢呈腺泡样结构。部分癌巢细胞发生坏死。（采煤工作 8 年，其他工作 8 年）（H.E 染色）

Fig.148 Coal workers' pneumoconiosis with pulmonary adenosquamous carcinoma: Besides coal dust cells foci, the lung showing adenosquamous carcinoma with regional necrosis that tumor cells form acinar structure and keratin reaction. (From the patient, working in coal mining ground service for 8 years respectively) (H.E stain)

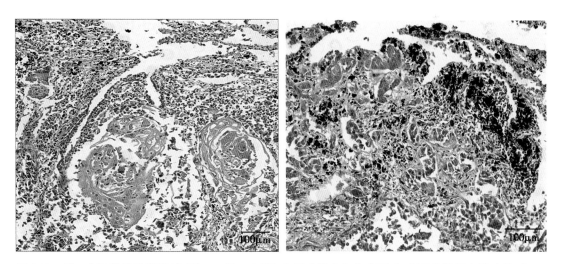

图 149 煤工尘肺伴发腺鳞癌（与图 148 同一病例）：左图癌巢中角化珠形成，右图腺管样癌巢形成。（H.E 染色）

Fig.149 Coal workers' pneumoconiosis with pulmonary adenosquamous carcinoma (sample is same as Fig.148): (Left) Keratin pears in tumor cell nests. (Right) Glandular structure of tumor cell nests. (H.E stain)

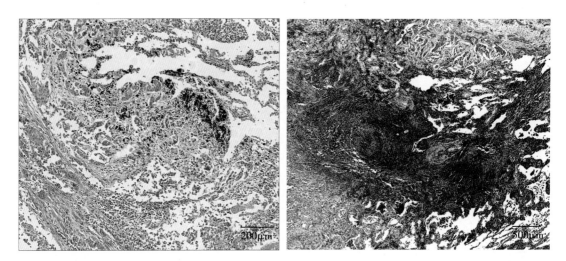

图 150　煤工尘肺伴发腺鳞癌（与图 148 同一病例）：左图显示肺内煤尘沉积，部分癌巢呈腺泡样结构，可见一些角化的细胞。右图显示煤尘纤维灶形成，周围的癌组织侵入病灶中。（H.E 染色）

Fig.150　Coal workers' pneumoconiosis with pulmonary adenosquamous carcinoma (sample is same as Fig.148): (Left) Microscopic view shows coal dust deposits mixed with carcinoma cells, which either arranges in the gland architecture or differentiates with keratin protein. (Right) Carcinoma tissue invasion of coal dust fibrous lesions. (H.E stain)

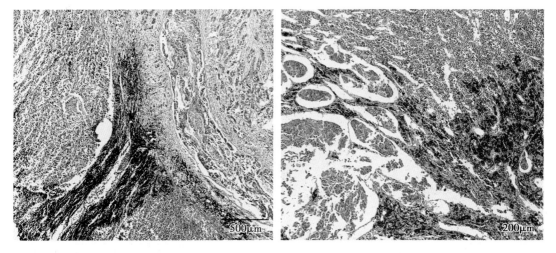

图 151　煤工尘肺伴发腺鳞癌（与图 148 同一病例）：左图显示支气管旁淋巴结转移，小静脉内癌栓形成，右图显示淋巴结内煤尘沉积，腺癌组织转移到肺门淋巴结内。（H.E 染色）

Fig.151　Coal workers' pneumoconiosis with pulmonary adenosquamous carcinoma (sample is same as Fig.148): (Left) Tumor cells are carried to the peribronchial lymph node, or small veins as tumor emboli. (Right) Both coal dust deposits and adenocarcinoma growth are seen in hilar lymph nodes. (H.E stain)

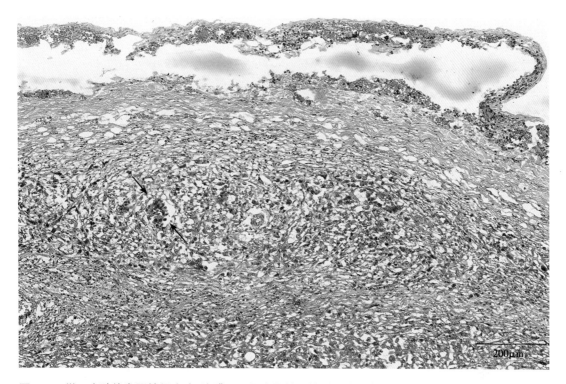

图 152 煤工尘肺伴发恶性间皮瘤：胸膜下可见弥漫性恶性间皮瘤细胞浸润，肿瘤细胞以具有肉瘤样特征的细胞为主，其中偶见上皮样肿瘤细胞灶（箭头）。（采煤工作 25 年）（H.E 染色）

Fig.152 Coal workers' pneumoconiosis with malignant mesothelioma: Diffuse subpleural invasion of malignant mesothelioma cells could be seen. The tumor cells predominantly show sarcomatous features with a few admixed epithelioid foci(Arrow). (From the patient, working in coal mining for 25 years) (H.E stain)

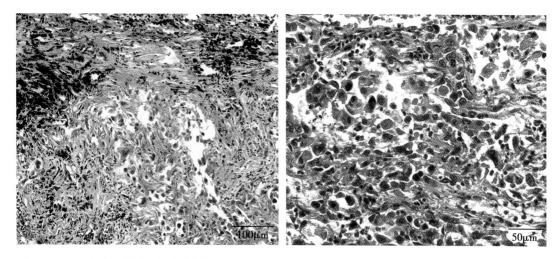

图 153 煤工尘肺伴发恶性间皮瘤（与图 152 同一病例）：左图显示较多煤尘沉积在肺内。其间可见大量弥漫浸润性生长的恶性瘤细胞，肺组织原有结构破坏，右图显示恶性异型的肿瘤细胞。（H.E 染色）

Fig.153 Coal workers' pneumoconiosis with malignant mesothelioma (sample is same as Fig.152): (Left) Numerous infiltrating malignant tumor cells, mixed with coal dust deposits, are diffusely distributed in lung, destroying the normal tissue. (Right) Malignant tumor cells with obvious atypia. (H.E stain)

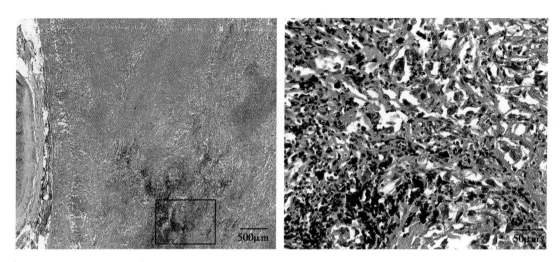

图 154　煤工尘肺伴发恶性间皮瘤淋巴结转移：支气管旁淋巴结内煤尘沉积。大量恶性瘤细胞弥漫浸润性生长，破坏了淋巴结组织原有结构。右图为左图局部放大。（与图 153 同一病例）（H.E 染色）

Fig.154　Coal workers' pneumoconiosis with lymph node malignant mesothelioma metastasis: Coal dust deposits in parbronchial lymph nodes. Abundant malignant tumor cells, characterized by diffuse infiltrating growth, destroy the residual tissue of lymph node. Right photography shows the details of high-power view. (Sample is same as Fig.153) (H.E stain)

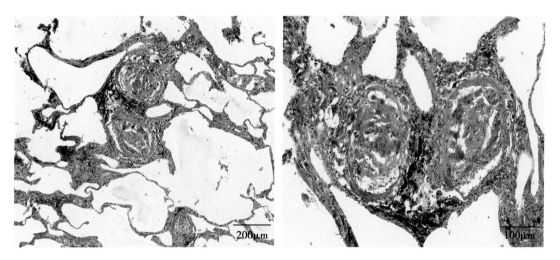

图 155　血管内瘤栓形成：肺内一些小血管扩张，其内可见恶性肿瘤细胞瘤栓形成。（与图 154 同一病例）（H.E 染色）

Fig.155　Carcinoma cells emboli in small blood vessels: The malignant tumor cells lodge in the dilated small blood vessels. (Sample is same as Fig.154) (H.E stain)

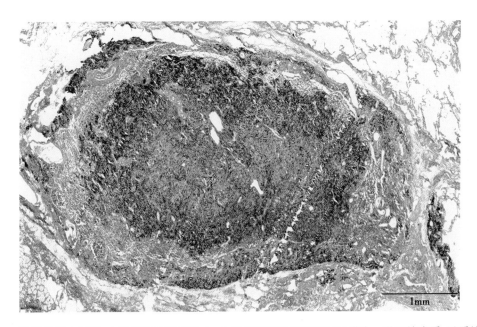

图156　淋巴结煤尘沉积:支气管旁淋巴结肿大、大量煤尘沉积伴纤维组织增生。淋巴结皮质、髓质结构尚清晰。(采煤、运煤20年)(H.E染色)
Fig.156　Lymph nodes with coal dust deposition: Abundant coal dust deposits and fibrous tissue in the enlarged peribronchial lymph node. Normal lymph node architecture is maintained at cortex. (From the patient, working in coal mining and transportation for 20 years) (H.E stain)

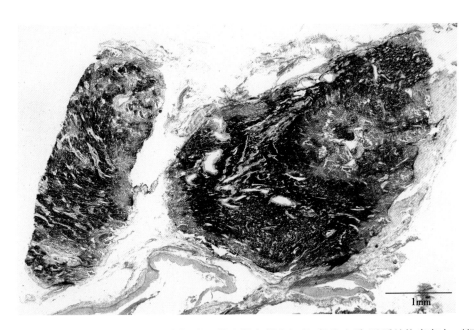

图157　淋巴结煤尘沉积:肺内淋巴结肿大,淋巴结内较多煤尘沉积,部分皮质、髓质结构尚存在。(掘进工作20年)(H.E染色)
Fig.157　Lymph nodes with coal dust deposition: A collection of numerous coal dust deposits in the enlarged pulmonary lymph nodes, note: cortex and medulla partially exist. (From the patient, working in coal tunneling for 20 years) (H.E stain)

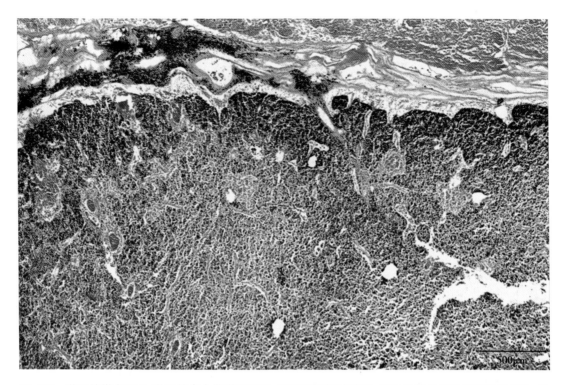

图 158 淋巴结煤尘沉积：淋巴结内大量煤尘沉积，淋巴结结构被破坏，仅保留部分原有的淋巴结结构，淋巴结被膜煤尘沉积、增厚。（采煤、掘进工作 17 年）（H.E 染色）

Fig.158 Lymph nodes with coal dust deposition: Low-power view revealing replacement of partial lymph node tissue by abundant coal dust deposits. The capsule is thickened. (From the patient, engaging on coal mining and tunneling for 17 years) (H.E stain)

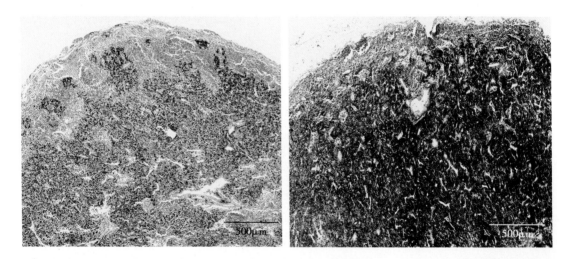

图 159 淋巴结煤尘沉积：淋巴结内较多煤尘沉积，原有淋巴结结构破坏。左图皮质区部分淋巴小结结构尚存留。（左图采煤、掘进工作 17 年，右图掘进工作 20 年）（H.E 染色）

Fig.159 Lymph nodes with coal dust deposition: Photography illustrating failure of lymph node, due to coal dust deposition. A patchy area of normal follicle structure is seen in the left image.〔From the patients, working in coal mining and tunneling for 17 years (left) and in coal tunneling for 20 years (right) 〕(H.E stain)

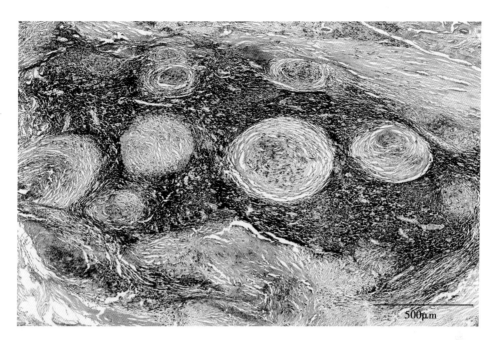

图 160　淋巴结内煤矽结节:淋巴结内多个煤矽结节形成。结节中央为"同心圆样"分布的胶原纤维,其外围是黑色煤尘沉积形成的"套袖样"结构环绕,原有淋巴结结构被破坏。(掘进工作 20 年)(H.E 染色)
Fig.160　Coal silicotic nodules in lymph nodes: Lymph node tissue is replaced by multiple coal silicotic nodules. A characteristic coal silicotic nodule reveals the central collagen in concentric circles of arrangement that is surrounded by the deposited coal dust, forming a "cuff-cover" appearance. (From the patient, working in coal tunneling for 20 years) (H.E stain)

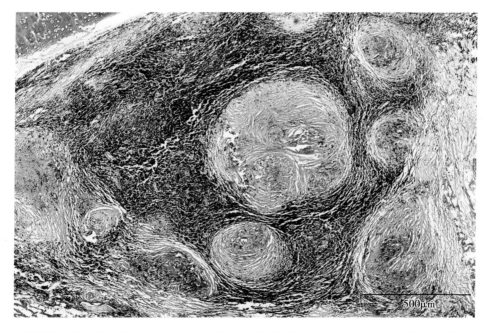

图 161　淋巴结内煤矽结节(与图 160 同一病例):支气管旁淋巴结内多个煤矽结节形成。(HE 染色)
Fig.161　Coal silicotic nodules in lymph nodes (sample is same as Fig.160): Multiple coal silicotic nodules are present at the peribronchial lymph node. (H.E stain)

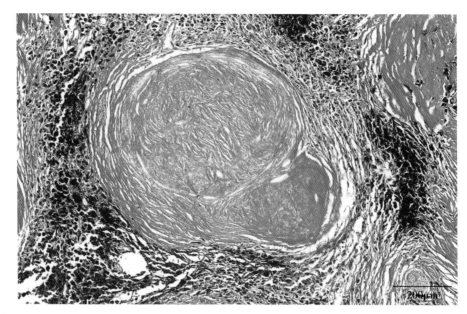

图 162　淋巴结内煤矽结节:玻璃样变性的胶原纤维呈"洋葱皮样"分布在结节中央,"套袖状"分布的煤尘沉积在结节外侧带。(井下测量工作 15 年)(H.E 染色)

Fig.162　Coal silicotic nodules in lymph nodes: Medium-power view illustrating the fibrous tissue with hyaline change, and collagen arranged in an onion-skin pattern, which forms the center of coal silicotic nodule, with a surrounding rim of coal dust deposits, looking like a "cuff-cover" appearance. (From the patient, working in underground survey for 15 years) (H.E stain)

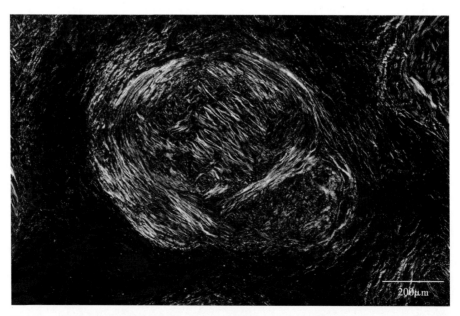

图 163　淋巴结内煤矽结节(与图 162 同一视野):结节内橙黄色为分布的I型胶原,绿色为分布的Ⅲ型胶原。(天狼猩红染色,偏振光观察)

Fig.163　Coal silicotic nodules in lymph nodes (same microscope field as Fig.162): Collagen type I is highlighted by orange, while collagen type III shows green. (Sirius red stain, polarized light microscopy with dark field)

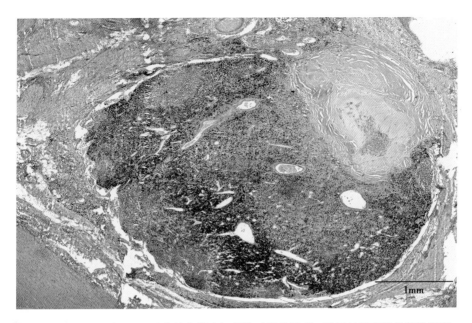

图 164 淋巴结病变：淋巴结内较多煤尘沉积伴矽结节形成。淋巴结原有结构部分保留。（掘进工作 9 年）（H.E 染色）

Fig.164 Silicotic lesions in lymph nodes: Partial lymph node tissue is replaced by coal dust deposits and silicotic nodules. (From the patient, working in coal tunneling for 9 years) (H.E stain)

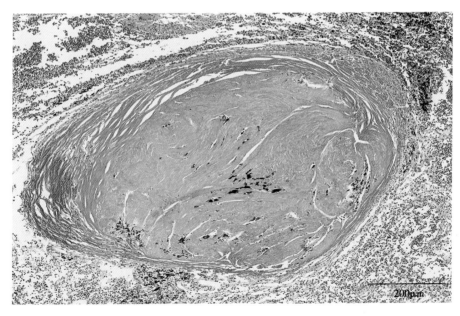

图 165 淋巴结内矽结节：结节中央胶原纤维发生玻璃样变性，外围胶原纤维呈"同心圆样"分布。少量煤尘沉积在结节内。（掘进工作 20 年）（H.E 染色）

Fig.165 Silicotic nodules in lymph node: Photography of silicotic nodule demonstrating the central collagen with hyaline change and the peripheral collagen in a concentric circles arrangement. Note minimal coal dust deposits in the silicotic nodule. (From the patient, working in coal tunneling for 20 years) (H.E stain)

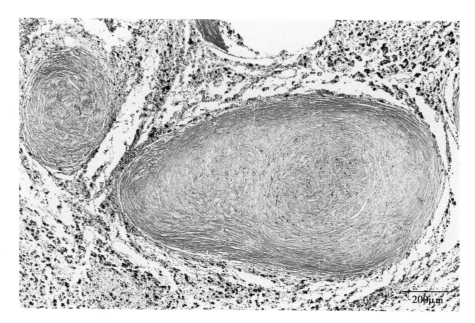

图 166 淋巴结内矽结节：结节内增生的胶原纤维呈"同心圆样"分布。(掘进工作 20 年)
(H.E 染色)

Fig.166　Silicotic nodules in lymph node: The proliferated fibrous tissue of nodules arranges in a concentric circles pattern. (From the patient, working in coal tunneling for 20 years) (H.E stain)

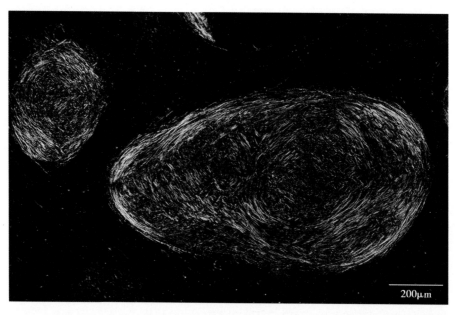

图 167 淋巴结矽结节(与图 166 同一视野)：结节内橙黄色为分布的 I 型胶原，绿色为分布的Ⅲ型胶原。(天狼猩红染色，偏振光观察)

Fig.167　Silicotic nodules in lymph node (same microscope field as Fig. 166): Collagen type I is stained with oranger, while collagen type III shows green. (Sirius red stain, polarized light microscopy with dark field)

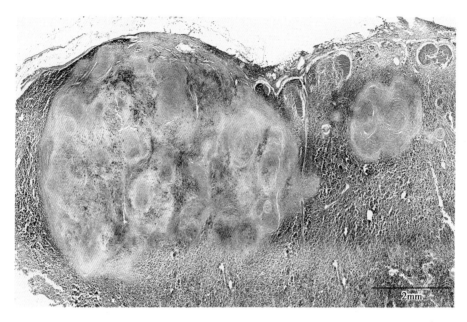

图 168 淋巴结内融合型矽结节：多个矽结节融合成一个较大结节。大量煤尘沉积在淋巴结内，原有淋巴结结构被破坏。（井下测量工作 15 年）（H.E 染色）

Fig.168 Confluent silicotic nodules in lymph node: Microscopic illustration of a large area of silicotic nodule, created by coalesces of several small ones, in the coal dust-deposited lymph node with normal tissue failure. (From the patient, working in underground survey for 15 years) (H.E stain)

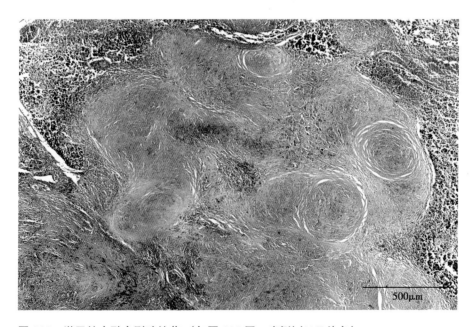

图 169 淋巴结内融合型矽结节。（与图 168 同一病例）（H.E 染色）

Fig.169 Confluent silicotic nodules in lymph node. (Sample is same as Fig.168) (H.E stain)

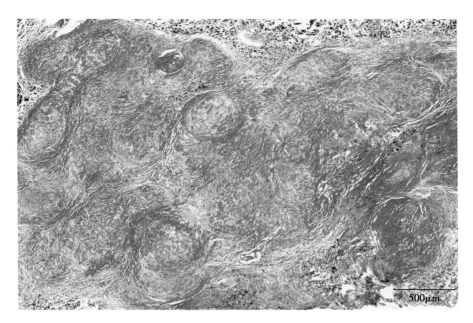

图 170　淋巴结内融合型矽结节（与图 168 同一病例）: 多个结节融合成较大的结节。结节内大量增生胶原纤维呈玻璃样变性（红色）。（天狼星红染色, 偏振光明场观察）

Fig.170　Confluent silicotic nodules in lymph node (Sample is same as Fig.168): Several silicotic nodules merge to form a massive nodule with hyaline dense collagen (red). (Sirius red stain, polarized light microscope with light field)

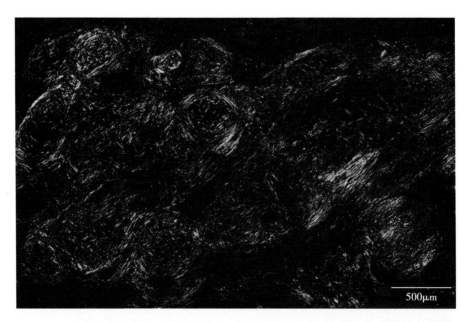

图 171　淋巴结内融合型矽结节（与图 170 同一视野）: 结节内橙黄色为Ⅰ型胶原, 绿色为Ⅲ型胶原。（天狼星红, 偏振光暗场）

Fig.171　Confluent silicotic nodules in lymph node (same microscope field as Fig 170): Collagen type I is highlighted by orange, while collagen type III shows green.(Sirius red stain, polarized light microscopy with dark field)

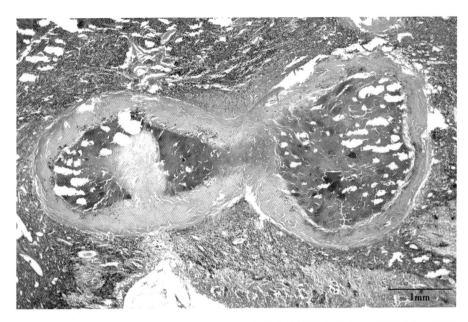

图172 淋巴结内煤矽结核结节:淋巴结内两个煤矽结核结节融合,中央区域发生坏死与钙化。(采煤工作22年)(H.E染色)

Fig.172 Coal silicotic tuberculous nodules in lymph nodes: Low-power view of lymph nodes reveals coalescence of two coal silicotic tuberculous nodules with central caseous necrosis and calcification response. (From the patient, working in coal mining for 22 years) (H.E stain)

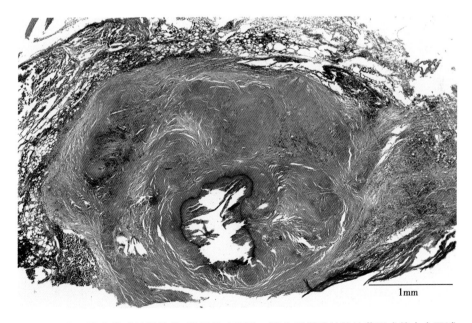

图173 淋巴结内煤矽结核结节:淋巴结内可见一融合型煤矽结核结节形成伴中央区域发生坏死与钙化。(岩凿工作20年)(H.E染色)

Fig.173 Coal silicotic tuberculous nodules in lymph nodes: A confluent coal silicotic tuberculous nodules with central necrosis and calcification, is visible in the lymph node. (From the patient, working in rock drilling for 20 years) (H.E stain)

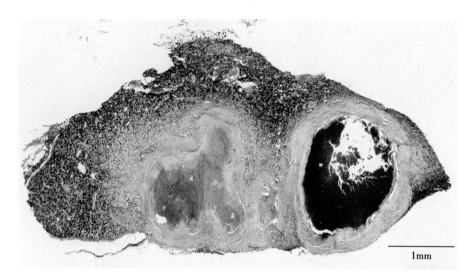

图 174　淋巴结内矽结核结节：淋巴结内两个矽结核结节融合，中央区域发生坏死与钙化，淋巴结原有结构被破坏。（采煤、掘进、井下运输 31 年）（H.E 染色）
Fig.174　Silicotic tuberculous nodules in lymph nodes: Microscopic illustration of coalescence of two coal silicotic tuberculosis nodules, which shows caseous necrosis and calcification in center. Note destruction of lymph node. (From the patient, working in coal mining, tunneling and transportation for 31 years) (H.E stain)

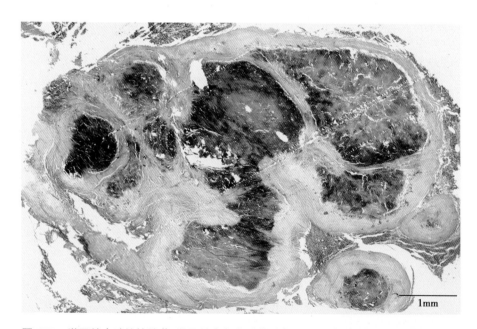

图 175　淋巴结内矽结核结节：淋巴结内多个结节融合，增生的纤维组织包饶在每个结节外围，中央区域发生坏死与钙化。融合型结节外侧煤尘沉积。（采煤工作 22 年）（H.E 染色）
Fig.175　Silicotic tuberculous nodules in lymph nodes: Low-power view of lymph nodes reveals coalescence of several silicotic tuberculous nodules, each of which is entrapped by the proliferated collagen with central necrosis and calcification, and coal dust deposition around the confluent nodules. (From the patient, working in coal mining for 22 years) (H.E stain)

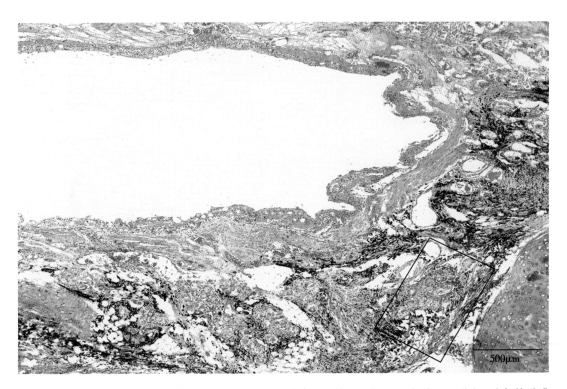

图 176　煤尘侵及支气管:大量煤尘沉积在支气管壁,壁内小血管增生与充血,纤维组织增生。支气管黏膜下层内的腺体被侵及、破坏。(采煤 4 年及其他混合工种 4 年)(H.E 染色)

Fig.176　Coal dust deposition in bronchi: Abundant coal dust deposits in the wall of bronchi with congested small blood vessels and fibrous proliferation. Mucous glands in submucosa are destroyed. (From the patient, performing on coal mining and other work for 4 years respectively) (H.E stain)

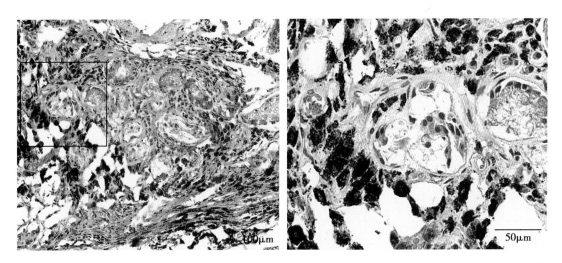

图 177　煤尘侵及支气管:左图为图 176 局部放大,大量煤尘沉积,伴纤维组织增生。支气管黏膜下层腺体被侵及、破坏;右图为左图局部放大。(H.E 染色)

Fig.177　Coal dust deposition in bronchi: Regional amplification of Fig.176 (left) and its details (right) illustrate the characteristic deposits of coal dust in the wall of bronchi. Note proliferation of fibrous tissue and destruction of glands in submucosa. (H.E stain)

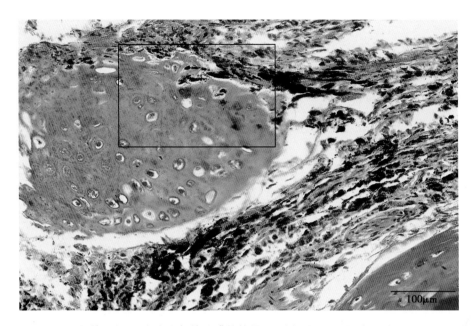

图 178　煤尘侵及支气管:煤尘沉积在支气管外膜的软骨间,伴纤维组织增生。局部可见煤尘伴增生的纤维组织突破软骨被膜,侵入软骨内。(采煤工作 4 年及其他混合工种 4 年)(H.E 染色)

Fig.178　Coal dust invasion into bronchi: Microscopic view of bronchi wall reveals coal dust deposition between cartilage plates. The proliferated fibrous tissue with coal dust deposits penetrates into cartilage capsule, involving the cartilage tissue. (From the patient, performing on coal mining and other work for 4 years respectively) (H.E stain)

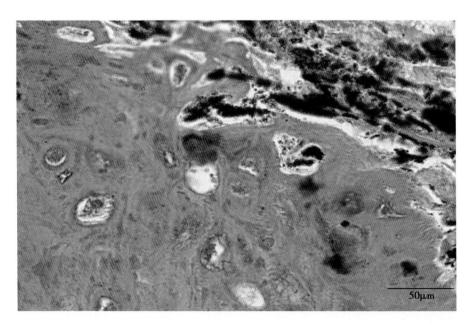

图 179　煤尘侵及支气管(图 178 局部放大):黑色的煤尘呈"虫蚀"状突破软骨被膜,并沉积在软骨陷窝内。(H.E 染色)

Fig.179　Coal dust invasion into bronchi (high-power view of Fig.178): Showing coal dust deposits penetrate into the cartilage capsule and deposit in the cartilage lacuna. (H.E stain)

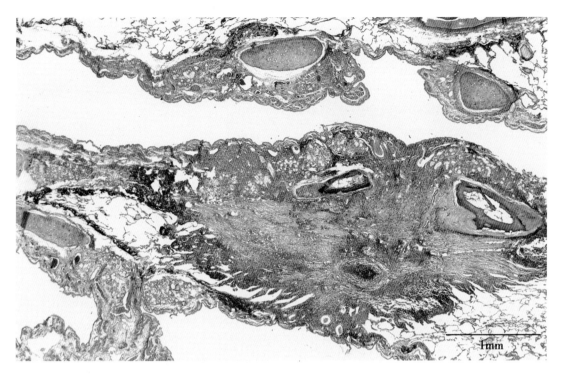

图 180　煤尘侵及支气管：支气管壁大量纤维组织灶状增生伴钙化。（采煤、井下运输工作 22 年）（H.E 染色）
Fig.180　Coal dust deposition in bronchi: Massive pattern of dense collogen and calcification response are visible in bronchial wall. (From the patient, working in coal mining and transportation for 22 years) (H.E stain)

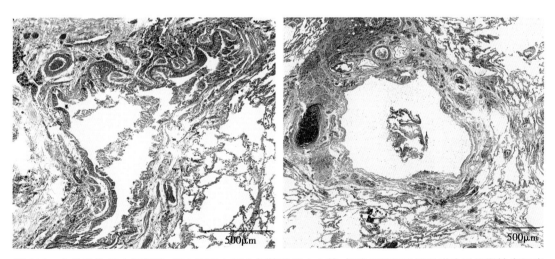

图 181　尘性慢性细支气管炎：煤尘沉积在细支气管壁伴小血管、纤维组织和平滑肌增生以及慢性炎细胞浸润，管腔内黏液栓形成。左图，尘性纤维组织挤压支气管壁呈迂曲花边状（井下测量工作 15 年）；右图，壁内黏液腺增生。（回采、掘进工作 17 年）（H.E 染色）
Fig.181　Coal chronic bronchiolitis: Coal dust accumulation in bronchiole wall containing the proliferated small vessels, collagen, smooth muscle cells and chronic inflammatory cells, with a mucous plug in lumen. Note a segment of the prilly wall, a consequence of compression of proliferted fibrous tissue (left); proliferated mucous glands of the bronchiole wall (right).〔From the patients, working in underground survey for 15 years (left) and in coal mining and tunneling for 17 years〕(H.E stain)

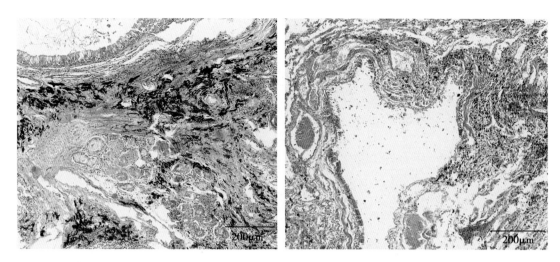

图 182 尘性慢性支气管炎:左图显示煤尘沉积在支气管壁伴纤维组织增生,包绕与破坏增生的腺体,右图显示支气管壁内慢性炎细胞浸润,局部支气管粘膜上皮脱落。(采煤工作 22 年)(H.E 染色)

Fig.182 Coal chronic bronchiolitis: Coal dust deposits in the wall of bronchioles, combined with dense collagen, encapsulation and destroy of the proliferated glands (Left). Chronic inflammatory cell infiltration in the bronchioles wall, accompanied with regional desquamation of epithelial cells of mucosa (Right). (From the patient, working in coal mining for 22 years) (H.E stain)

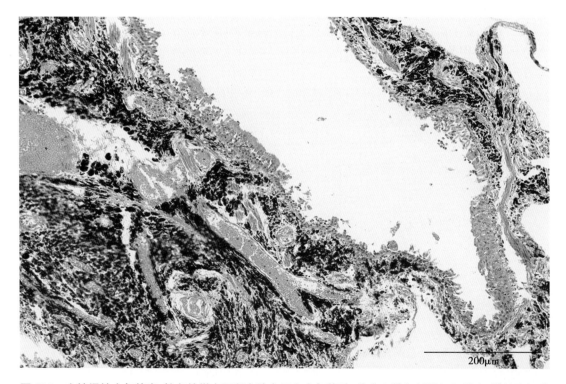

图 183 尘性慢性支气管炎:较多的煤尘沉积在肺内细小支气管壁,伴小血管与纤维组织增生,慢性炎细胞浸润。局部支气管鳞状上皮化生。(采煤工作 22 年)(H.E 染色)

Fig.183 Coal chronic bronchiolitis: Abundant coal dust deposits in the wall of bronchioles, with proliferation of small vessels, collagen and infiltration of chronic inflammatory cells. Note squamous metaplasia in mucosa. (From the patient, working in coal mining for 22 years) (H.E stain)

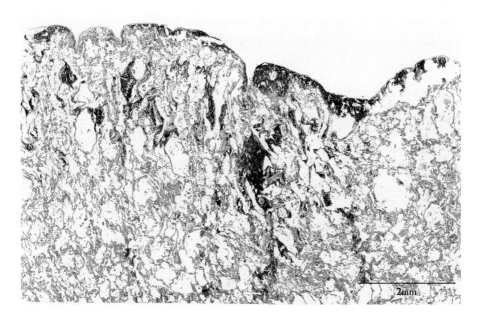

图 184 胸膜病变：煤尘聚集在胸膜，使胸膜局部增厚。胸膜下方煤尘灶形成，似"泪滴"状分布在胸膜下方的肺组织中。（采煤、掘进、井下运输工作 31 年）（HE 染色）

Fig.184 Pleural lesions: Moderate amount of coal dust deposits in pleura results in pleural thickening. Coal dust foci under the pleura distribute in a "tear dropping" pattern. (From the patient, working in coal mining, tunneling and transportation for 31 years) (H.E stain)

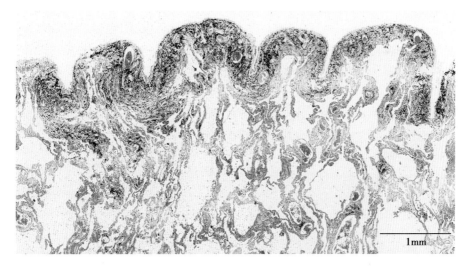

图 185 胸膜病变：煤尘聚集在胸膜，伴纤维组织与小血管增生，使增厚的胸膜似"城墙垛"向表面凸出。胸膜下方肺组织间质纤维化、小血管增生，部分肺泡腔扩张。（采煤、掘进工作 17 年）（H.E 染色）

Fig.185 Pleural lesions: The thickening pleura containg coal dusts deposits, proliferated collagen fibers and small blood vessles resembles "city battlements", associated with interstitial fibrosis, small vessel proliferation and regional airspace dilation in subplerual pulmonary tissue. (From the patient, working in coal mining and tunneling for 17 years) (H.E stain)

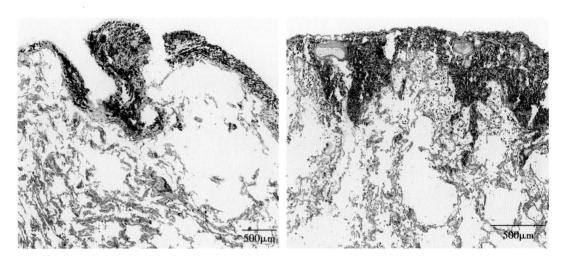

图 186　胸膜病变：较多煤尘聚集胸膜，伴随纤维组织增生与小血管增生，使胸膜增厚。左图，增厚的胸膜呈"息肉"状向胸膜表面凸出，胸膜直下伴肺气肿形成（采煤、掘进工作 11 年）；右图，增厚的胸膜似"树根"状沿着肺间质向下伸延。（采煤、掘进工作 15 年）（H.E 染色）

Fig.186　Pleural lesions: Coal dusts deposition, combined with collagen and small blood vessles, results in pleura thickening. Note a polyp-shaped thickening lesion projecting to the surface of pleura, with subplerual emphysema formation (left); the thickening lesions also extending along pulmonary interstitial tissue, like "spike" (right).〔From the patients, working in coal mining and tunneling for 11 years (left) and 15 years (right)〕(H.E stain)

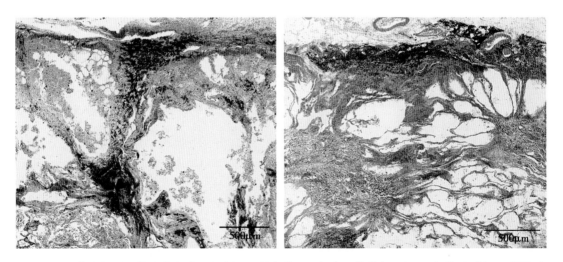

图 187　胸膜病变：煤尘聚集在胸膜及小叶间隔，伴纤维组织与小血管增生。左图，胸膜、小叶间隔增厚，胸膜下方部分肺泡腔扩张，内含炎性渗出物；右图，增生纤维组织向下伸延与胸膜下方形成的非典型纤维性结节相连在一起。（采煤工作 21 年）（H.E 染色）

Fig187　Pleural lesions: Coal dust accumulation in pleura and interlobular septum, accompanied with proliferation of collagen and small vessels. Left photography also illustrating a thicking of pleura and interlobular septum, with inflammatory exsudates in lumen of partial dialated airspace. Right image showing the junction of the subplerual atypical fibrous nodules and the pleural proliferated collagen which extends along pulmonary interstitial tissue. (From the patient, working in coal mining for 21 years) (H.E stain)

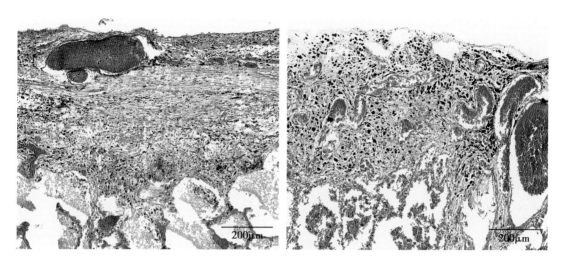

图 188　胸膜病变:胸膜内煤尘沉积伴纤维组织增生,胸膜明显增厚,其内小血管增生伴血栓形成。(左图掘进工作 17 年,右图回采、掘进工作 17 年)(H.E 染色)

Fig.188　Pleural lesions: The thickening pleura contains coal dust deposits, dense collagen and proliferated small vessels with thrombosis.〔From the patients, working in coal tunneling for 17 years (left) and in coal mining and tunneling for 17 years (right)〕(H.E stain)

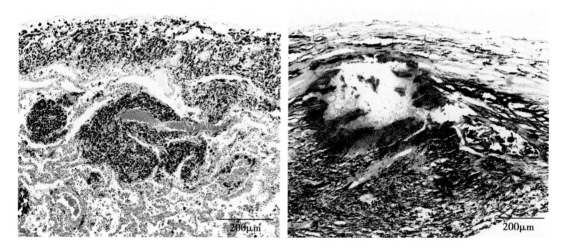

图 189　胸膜病变:煤尘聚集在胸膜,伴纤维组织增生,胸膜增厚,局部胸膜发生钙化。胸膜下方煤尘细胞性结节形成。(采煤、掘进工作 17 年)(HE 染色)

Fig.189　Pleural lesions: The thickening pleura reveals coal dust deposits, prolifetated fibrous tissue and abnormal deposition of calcium salts. Note cellular coal dust nodules in subpleural pulmonary tissue. (From the patient, working in coal mining and tunneling for 17 years) (H.E stain)

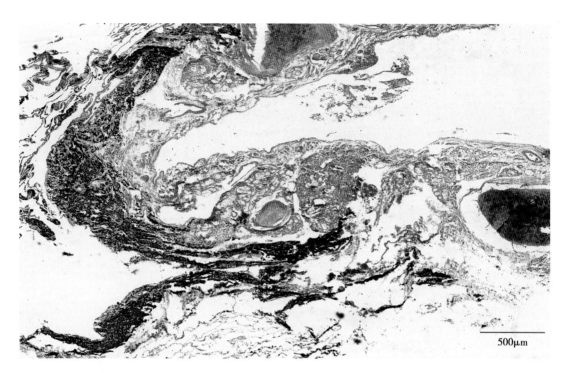

图 190　煤尘沉积在肺内小支气管:煤尘沉积于肺内小支气管管壁,伴纤维组织增生,炎细胞浸润,支气管壁增厚。(采煤、掘进工作 11 年)(HE 染色)

Fig.190　Coal dust deposition in small bronchia: Microscopic view of small bronchia demonstrating the thicking wall, containing aboudant coal dust deposits, proliferated collagen and infiltrated chronic inflammatory cells. (From the patient, working in coal mining and tunneling for 11 years) (H.E stain)

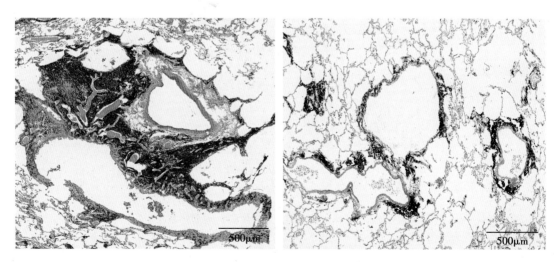

图 191　煤尘沉积在肺内细支气管及终末细支气管:左图,较多的煤尘沉积在肺内细支气管壁一侧,伴小血管和纤维组织增生;右图,煤尘沉积在肺内细支气管及终末细支气管。(采煤工作 22 年)(H.E 染色)

Fig.191　Coal dust deposition in small bronchia and terminal bronchia: (Left) Moderate amount of coal dust accumulation in a segment of small bronchia wall, accompanied with proliferation of collagen and small vessels. (Right) Minimal coal dust depostion in the wall of small bronchia and terminal bronchia. (From the patient, working in coal mining for 22 years) (H.E stain)

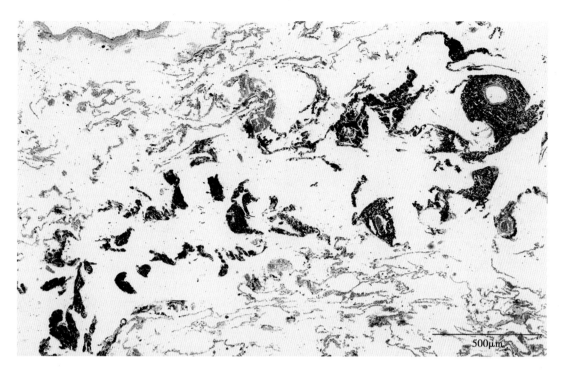

图 192 煤尘沉积在呼吸性细支气管及其分支：煤尘沿着呼吸性细支气管、肺泡管、肺泡囊沉积，伴随着煤尘细胞灶及细胞性结节形成。（采煤、掘进工作 11 年）（H.E 染色）

Fig.192 Coal dust deposition in respiratory bronchia and its branaches: Photomicrograghy illustration of coal dust deposition along the respiratory bronchia, alveolar ducts and alveolar sacs, with formation of coal dust cell foci and coal cellular nodules. (From the patient, working in coal mining and tunneling for 11 years) (H.E stain)

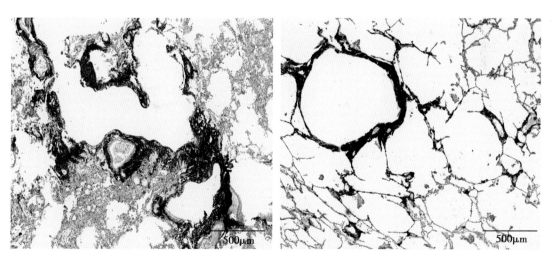

图 193 煤尘沉积在呼吸性细支气管及其分支：煤尘沿着呼吸性细支气管、肺泡管、肺泡腔沉积，伴小气道和肺泡腔的扩张。（掘进工作 20 年）（H.E 染色）

Fig.193 Coal dust deposition in respiratory bronchia and its branaches: Coal dust deposition along the respiratory bronchia, alveolar ducts and alveolar sacs, with dilation of small airway and airspace. (From the patient, working in coal tunneling for 20 years) (H.E stain)

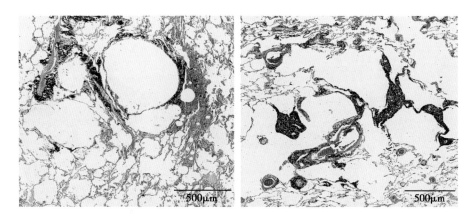

图 194 尘性小叶中心型肺气肿：煤尘沿着呼吸性细支气管沉积，伴随着煤斑（左图，掘进工 20 年）、煤尘灶（右图，回采和掘进工作 17 年）和小叶中心型肺气肿形成。（H.E 染色）

Fig.194 Coal dust-induced centriacinar emphysema: Photomicrograghy illustration of coal dust deposition around respiratory bronchia, with fomation of coal dust dots (left), coal dust foci (right) and centriacinar emphysema.〔From the patients, working in coal tunneling for 20 years (left) and in coal mining and tunneling for 17 years (right)〕 (H.E stain)

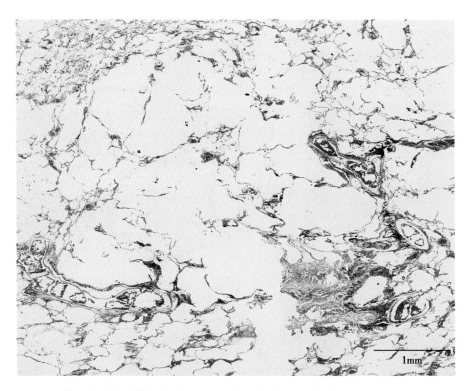

图 195 全小叶破坏型肺气肿：煤尘沉积伴全小叶破坏型肺气肿形成。（回采和掘进工作 17 年）（H.E 染色）

Fig.195 Destructive panacinar emphysema: Coal dust deposition with destructive panacinar emphysema. (From the patient, working in coal mining and tunneling for 17 years) (H.E stain)

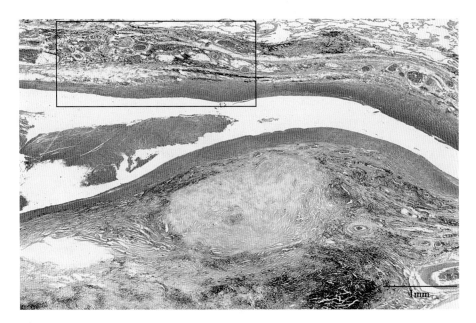

图 196 累及肺动脉：肺动脉一侧矽结节形成，挤压动脉壁，动脉腔狭窄。另一侧煤尘沉积在动脉壁外侧，伴小血管和纤维组织增生。（采煤和掘进工作 17 年）（H.E 染色）
Fig.196 Lesions in pulmonary artery: Pulmonary artery is sectioned longitudinally to reveal narrowing of lumen, due to compression of silicotic nodules in one side of the wall. Coal dust also deposits in the opposite side, with proliferation of small blood vessels and collagen. (From the patient, working in coal mining and tunneling for 17 years) (H.E stain)

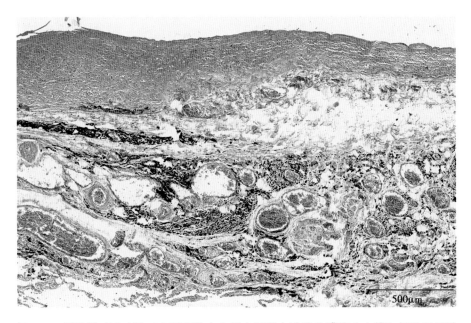

图 197 累及肺动脉：(图 196 局部放大)：煤尘沉积在动脉外膜伴小血管和纤维组织增生，煤尘侵入到动脉的平滑肌层。(H.E 染色)
Fig.197 Lesions in pulmonary artery (regional amplification of Fig. 196): Photography of pulmonary artery showing a collection of coal dust in adventitia, with proliferation of small blood vessels and collagen. Note invasion of coal dust to the media. (H.E stain)

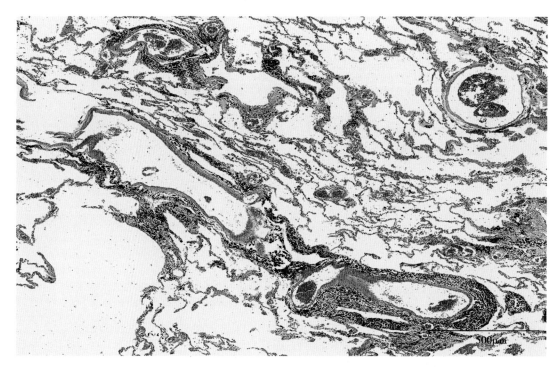

图 198　肺内小动脉病变:较多煤尘呈"套袖样"围绕肺内小动脉沉积。(采煤和掘进工作 11 年)(H.E 染色)
Fig.198　Lesions in pulmonary small arteries: Moderate amount of coal dust encloses the small arteries in a "cuff-cover" pattern. (From the patient, working in coal mining and tunneling for 11 years) (H.E stain)

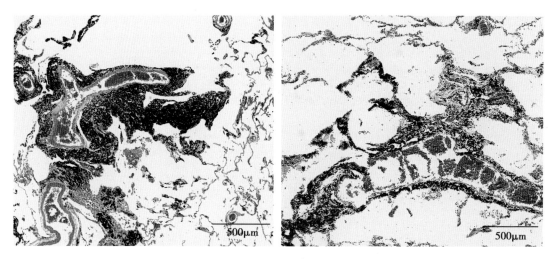

图 199　肺内小血管病变:左图显示小动脉的累及。大量煤尘呈"套袖样"包裹在小动脉外侧伴纤维组织增生,形成细胞纤维灶(采煤和掘进工作 11 年);右图显示小静脉的病变。煤尘呈"套袖样"包裹在肺内小静脉周围,一些煤尘沉积在邻近的肺泡壁。(掘进工作 20 年)(H.E 染色)
Fig.199　Lesions in pulmonary small vessels: (Left) Pulmonary small arteries are enclosed by a large amount of coal dust deposits in a sleevelet pattern, a consequence of cellular fibrotic foci formation. (Right) Coal dust also deposits around small veins (a sleevelet appearance), or in the adjacent alveolar septum. 〔From the patiens, working in coal mining and tunneling working for 11 years (left) and in coal tunneling for 20 years (right) 〕(H.E stain)

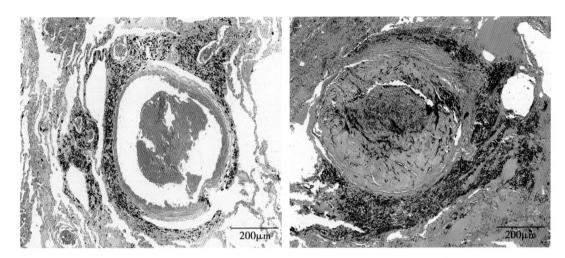

图 200 小动脉病变:左图显示,煤尘呈"套袖样"包裹在肺内小动脉外侧,局部侵入小动脉壁平滑肌层,动脉腔内血栓形成(采煤和掘进工作 11 年);右图显示肺小动脉壁平滑肌增生伴血栓形成并机化,煤尘呈"套袖样"沉积在动脉壁外侧,并侵入动脉壁各层及血栓内。(岩掘工作 7 年)(H.E 染色)

Fig.200 Lesions in small arteries: (Left) Photography of small artery showing a collection of coal dust in adventitia (a "cuff-cover" appearance) and local invasion to media, with an embolus in lumen. (Right) A small artery with an organized embolus shows reduplication of smooth muscle cells. Note coal dust deposits around the small blood vessels (a "cuff-cover" appearance), some of which invades to the entire wall and embolus.〔From the patient, working in coal mining and tunneling working for 11 years (left) and in rock drilling for 7 years (right)〕(H.E stain)

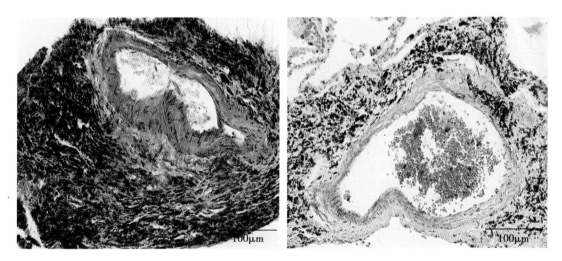

图 201 小动脉病变:煤尘呈"套袖样"包裹在肺内小动脉外侧,局部侵入小动脉壁平滑肌层。左图显示形成煤尘细胞性结节(掘进工作 20 年);右图显示动脉腔内血栓形成,血管腔内可见血细胞间夹杂煤尘颗粒。(采煤和掘进工作 11 年)(H.E 染色)

Fig.201 Lesions in the pulmonary small artery: A large amount of coal dust encloses the pulmonary small artery in a "cuff-cover" pattern, with local invasion to smooth muscle cell layer. Note the involved small vessels also showing cellular coal dust nodule formation (left), or coal dust deposits combined with blood cells and thrombus formation in lumen (right).〔From the patients, working in coal tunneling working for 20 years (left) and in coal mining and tunneling for 11 years (right)〕(H.E stain)

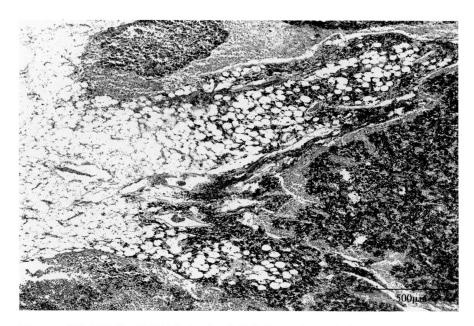

图 202　煤尘累及淋巴结及其脂肪组织：大量煤尘沉积在淋巴结中，并侵及周围的脂肪组织中。(井下机电维修工作 20 年)(H.E 染色)

Fig.202　Coal dust deposits involve lymph nodes and adipose tissue: A large amount of coal dust deposits in the lymph nodes, spreading to the surrounding adipose tissue. (From the patient, working in underground maintenance of equipment and electricity for 20 years) (H.E stain)

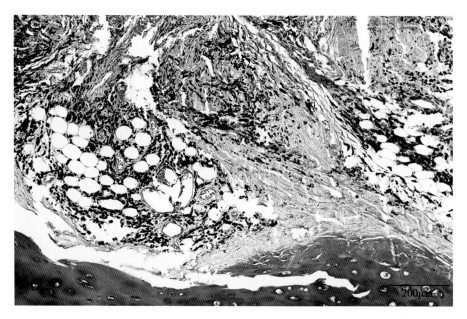

图 203　煤尘累及支气管及其周围脂肪组织。大量煤尘沉积在支气管外膜伴纤维组织增生，同时煤尘侵及周围的脂肪组织。(采煤 4 年及其他混合工种 4 年)(H.E 染色)

Fig.203　Involvement of bronchi and adjacent fat tissue by coal dusts: A heavy deposition of coal dust is visible in the adventitia of bronchi with dense collagen, and the surrounding fat tissue. (From the patient, performing on coal mining and other work for 4 years respectively) (H.E stain)

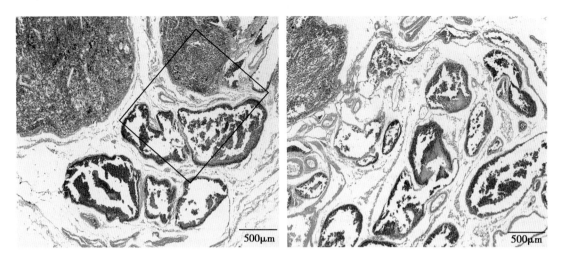

图204 淋巴管病变：淋巴结旁淋巴管扩张，较多煤尘沉积在淋巴管管壁与淋巴管管腔内。（掘进工作20年）（H.E染色）

Fig.204 Lesions in the lymphatic vessels: Moderate amount of coal dust deposits are present at both wall and lumen of the dilated lymphatic vessels next to the lymph nodes. (From the patient, working in coal tunneling working for 20 years) (H.E stain)

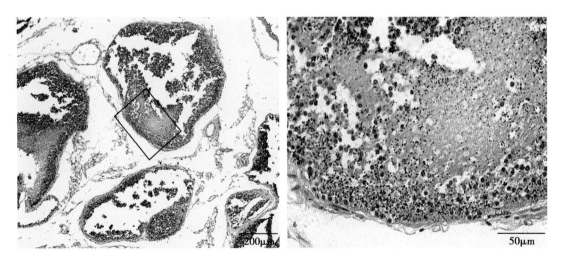

图205 淋巴管病变：左图为上图局部放大，右图为左图局部放大。

Fig.205 Lesions in the lymphatic vessels: (Left) Regional amplification of Fig. 204. (Right) Local details of the left one.

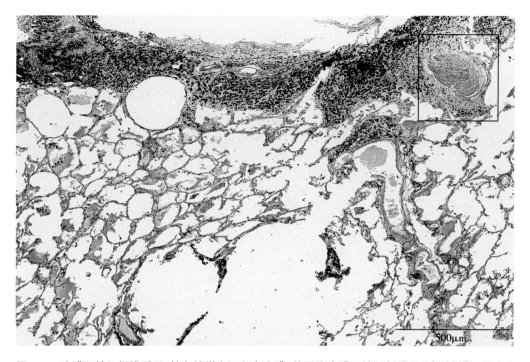

图206 胸膜下神经纤维受累：较多的煤尘沉积在胸膜，并围绕胸膜下神经纤维呈"套袖样"沉积。(采煤、掘进工作 29 年)(H.E 染色)

Fig.206 Coal dusts involve subpleural nerve fibers: Moderate amount of coal dust deposits in pleura and around the subpleural nerve fibers in a "cuff-cover" pattern. (From the patient, working in coal mining and tunneling for 29 years) (H.E stain)

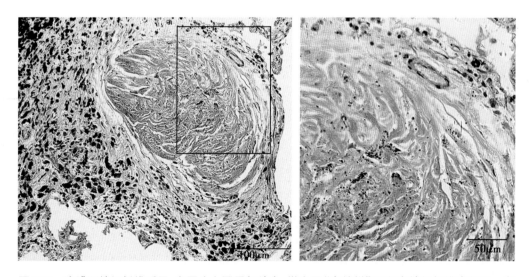

图 207 胸膜下神经纤维受累：左图为上图局部放大，煤尘呈"套袖样"沉积在神经纤维束周围。右图为左图局部放大，显示煤尘侵入神经纤维内。(H.E 染色)

Fig.207 Coal dust involved subpleural nerve fibers: (Left) A detail of Fig 204, showing coal dust accumulation around the nerve fibers in a sleevelet pattern. (Right) Focal amplification of the left photography, illustrating invasion of coal dust to nerve fibers. (H.E stain)

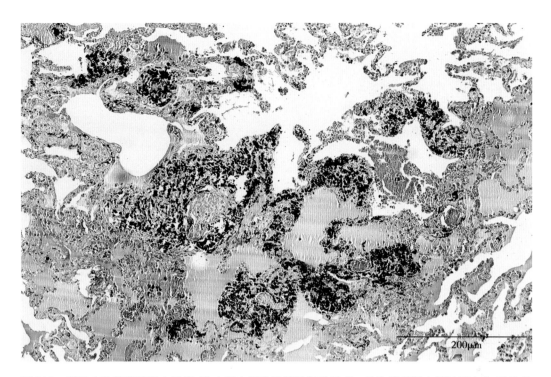

图208　煤工尘肺伴浆液出血性炎:肺内煤尘细胞灶伴肺气肿形成。肺泡壁毛细血管扩张充血,肺泡腔内含大量浆液性渗出物与漏出的红细胞。(掘进工作20年)(H.E染色)

Fig.208　Coal workers' pneumoconiosis with serous hemorrhagic inflammation: Cellular coal dust foci and emphysema action are visible in lung. Capillaries of alveolar septum are dilated; serous exudates and blood red cells are present at alveolar space. (From the patient, working in coal tunneling for 20 years) (H.E stain)

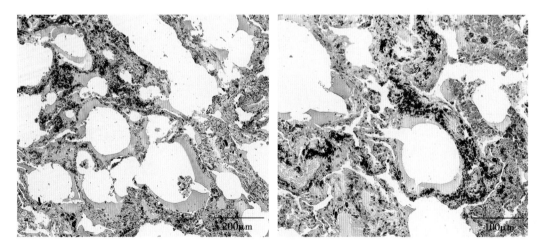

图209　煤工尘肺伴肺水肿:浆液渗出于肺泡腔内伴肺泡腔内透明膜形成。(掘进和采煤工作29年)(H.E染色)

Fig.209　Coal workers' pneumoconiosis with pulmonary edema: Alveolar spaces are lined by pink hyaline membranes, with collection of serous effusion. (From the patient, working in coal tunneling and mining for 29 years) (H.E stain)

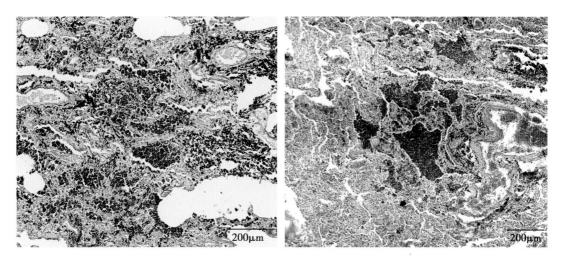

图 210　煤工尘肺伴肺淤血、肺水肿：肺组织中浆液渗出物伴淤血，肺泡腔内可见大量"心力衰竭细胞"。（掘进和采煤工作 29 年）（H.E 染色）

Fig.210　Coal workers' pneumoconiosis with pulmonary congestion and edema: Photography illustration of serous exudation and congestion response in lung, evidenced by congested small veins and abundant "heart failure" cells in alveolar spaces. (From the patient, working in coal tunneling and mining for 29 years) (H.E stain)

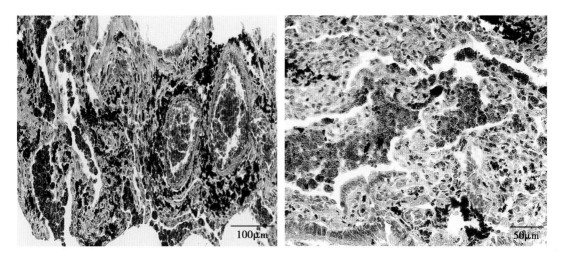

图 211　煤工尘肺伴肺淤血、肺水肿（与图 210 同一病例）：肺内小动脉充血，煤尘围绕小血管呈"套袖样"沉积。肺泡壁与肺泡腔内可见大量"心力衰竭细胞"。（H.E 染色）

Fig.211　Coal workers' pneumoconiosis with pulmonary congestion and edema (sample is same as Fig.210): Coal dust deposits enclose the congested small arteries in a "cuff-cover" pattern. Abundant "heart failure" cells are seen in alveolar septum and space. (H.E stain)

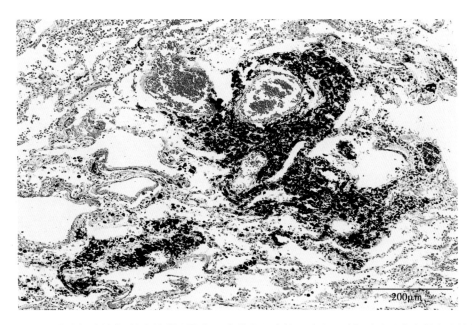

图 212　煤工尘肺伴化脓性炎：较多的煤尘聚集形成煤尘细胞灶。肺泡隔壁与肺泡腔内有较多中性粒细胞渗出，局部小血管扩张充血。（采煤工作 21 年）(H.E 染色）

Fig.212　Coal workers pneumoconiosis with purulent inflammation: Collection of moderate amount of coal dust responses to cellular coal dust foci. Note infiltrate of neutrophils in alveolar septum and space, dilation of small blood vessels. (From the patient, working in coal mining for 21 years) (H.E stain)

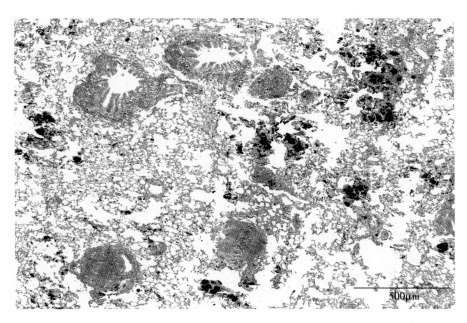

图 213　煤工尘肺伴脓肿：煤尘沉积在肺内小气道与肺泡腔，伴化脓性支气管炎和多发性微脓肿形成。（掘进工作 29 年）(H.E 染色）

Fig.213　Coal workers' pneumoconiosis with abscess: Coal dust deposition in the small airways and alveolar space, with suppurative bronchitis and multiple microabscesses. (From the patient, working in tunneling for 29 years) (H.E stain)

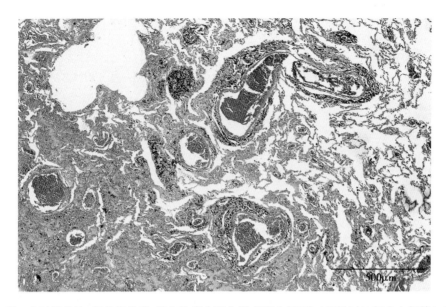

图 214　煤工尘肺伴浆液、纤维素性炎：较多的煤尘聚集形成煤尘（细胞／纤维）灶，细小支气管与肺泡腔内充填较多浆液、纤维素样渗出物，局部小血管扩张充血。（掘进、采煤工作 17 年）（H.E 染色）

Fig.214　Coal workers' pneumoconiosis with serous fibrinous inflammation: Moderate amount of coal dust deposits create either cellular coal dust foci or fibrous coal dust foci. Small bronchia and alveolar spaces are filled with serous exudates and fibrin, with vessel dilation and congestion. (From the patient, working in tunneling and coal mining for 17 years) (H.E stain)

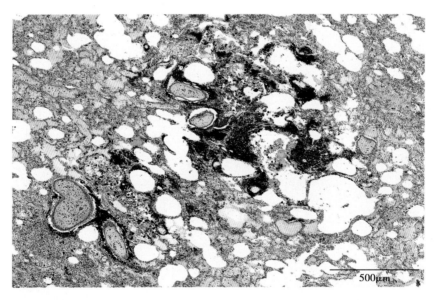

图 215　煤工尘肺伴浆液、化脓性炎：较多煤尘聚集形成煤尘（细胞／纤维）灶，周围肺泡腔内浆液和脓性渗出物充填。（采煤工作 21 年）（H.E 染色）

Fig.215　Coal workers' pneumoconiosis with serous purulent inflammation: Moderate amount of coal dust deposits create either cellular coal dust foci or fibrous coal dust foci, with the surrounding consolidated alveoli filled with serous exudates and purulent exudates. (From the patient, working in coal mining for 21 years) (H.E stain)

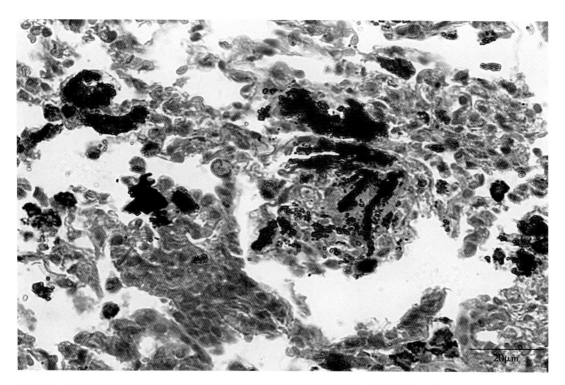

图 216　煤工尘肺"棒状小体"形成：肺泡腔与肺泡壁煤尘细胞聚集，多个"棒状小体"形成，伴肺泡上皮细胞增生。（掘进工作 20 年）（H.E 染色）

Fig.216　"Rod-shaped" bodies of coal workers' pneumoconiosis: High-power view illustration of rod-shaped" bodies, a consequence of coal dust-laden macrophages accumulation in alveolar septum and alveolar spaces, with alveolar epithelial cells proliferation. (From the patient, working in coal tunneling for 20 years) (H.E stain)

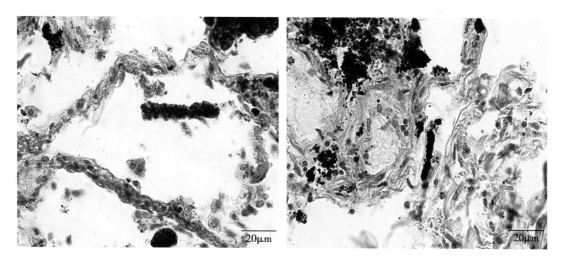

图 217　煤工尘肺"棒状小体"形成（与图 216 同一病例）：棒状小体游离于肺泡腔内。（HE 染色）

Fig.217　"Rod-shaped" bodies of coal workers' pneumoconiosis (sample is same as Fig. 216): "Rod-shaped" bodies are floating in alveolar space. (H.E stain)

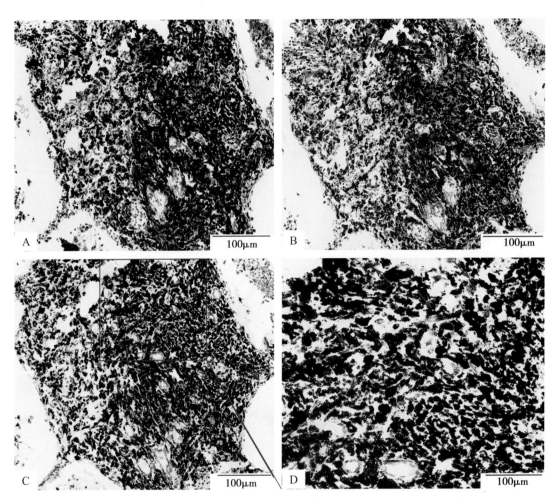

图 218　肌成纤维细胞分化：煤尘细胞性结节内可见大量煤尘沉积，伴少量纤维组织增生（A：H.E 染色；B：Masson 染色，煤尘细胞间蓝色的条索状结构为胶原纤维）。煤尘细胞间可见一些长梭形，多角形的细胞（箭头所指），胞浆着染棕黄色，为肌成纤维细胞（C：α-SMA 免疫组化染色，D：为左图的局部放大。（采煤工作 22 年）

Fig.218　Myofibroblasts differentiation: A, H.E section shows cellular coal dust nodules with abundant coal dust deposits and minimal fibrous tissue. B, Masson stain to accentuate the collagen (blue) between coal dust-laden macrophages. C and D (regional amplification of C), Immunoreactivity for α-smooth muscle actin (α-SMA) confirms the spindle or polygonal cells in the nodules are myofibroblasts. (From the patient, working in coal mining for 22 years)

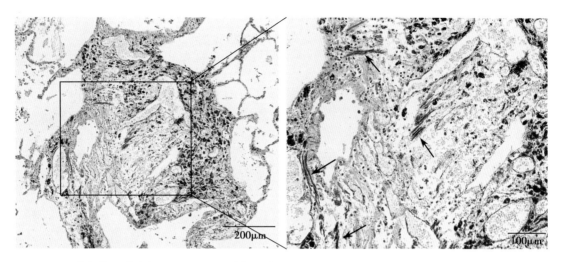

图 219 肌成纤维细胞分化：α-SMA 强阳性表达的细胞分布在早期细胞性结节中。右图为左图局部区域的放大。（采煤工作 4 年，井上其他工作 4 年）（α-SMA 免疫组织化学染色）

Fig.219 Myofibroblast differentiation: Left photography and its detail (right), show minimal cells with α-SMA strongly positive expression distributed in the early stage of cellular coal dust nodules. (From the patient, working in coal mining and ground service for 4 years respectively) (α-SMA immunohistochemical stain)

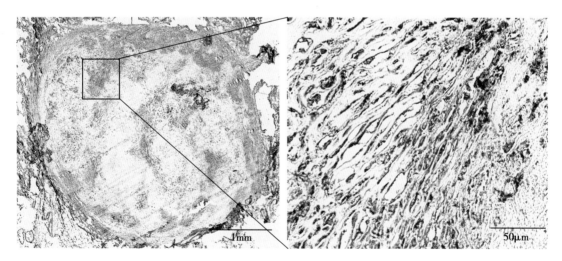

图 220 肌成纤维细胞分化：有较多 α-SMA 强阳性表达的细胞分布在煤工尘肺的矽（煤）结节内。右图为左图局部区域的放大。（井下测量工作 15 年）（α-SMA 免疫组织化学染色）

Fig.220 Myofibroblast differentiation: There are moderate amount of cells with strongly positively expression of α-SMA in silicotic (coal) nodules, shown in left image and its higher power view (right). (From the patient, working in underground survey for 15 years) (α-SMA immunohistochemical stain)

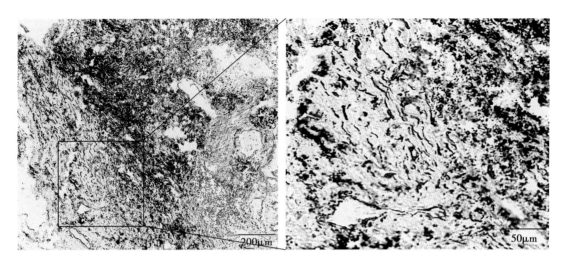

图 221　肌成纤维细胞分化：大量煤尘沉积在肺内伴弥漫性间质纤维化形成。在煤尘沉积的纤维化区域内可见较多 α-SMA 强阳性表达的肌成纤维细胞的分布。(掘进、井下运输 22 年)(α-SMA 免疫组织化学染色)
Fig.221　Myofibroblast differentiation: Abundant coal dust deposits in lung with diffuse interstitial fibrosis. Moderate cells with strongly positively expression of α-SMA are visible in the fibrous area with coal dust deposits (From the patient, working in coal tunneling and transportion for 22 years) (α-SMA immunohistochemical stain)

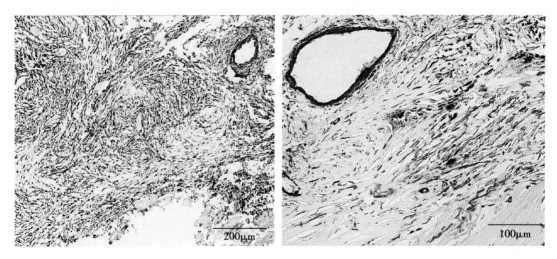

图 222　肌成纤维细胞分化：较多 α-SMA 强阳性表达的细胞分布在煤工尘肺的间质纤维化区域。(采煤工作 21 年)(α-SMA 免疫组织化学染色)
Fig.222　Myofibroblast differentiation: Moderate amount of cells with strongly positively expression of α-SMA are found in the fibrotic interstitial tissue, shown in left image and its higher power view (right). (From the patient, working in coal mining for 21 years) (α-SMA immunohistochemical stain)

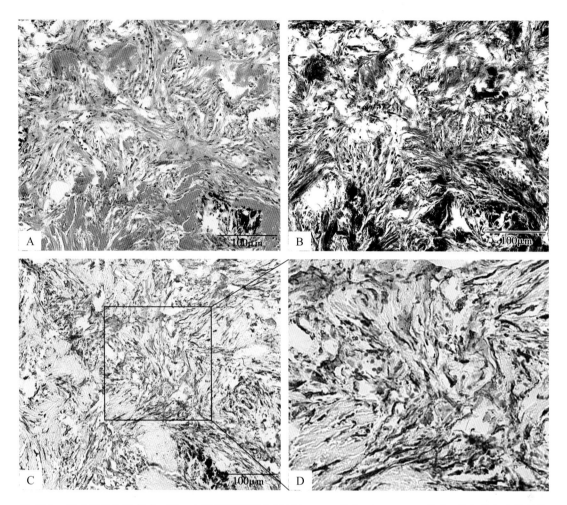

图 223 肌成纤维细胞分化:煤工尘肺间质纤维化区域(A:H.E 染色;B:Masson 染色,蓝色的条索状结构为胶原纤维)。(C:α-SMA 免疫组化染色,间质纤维化区域内有诸多长梭形,多角形胞浆着染棕黄色的肌成纤维细胞;D:为左图的局部放大。(凿岩工作 22 年)

Fig.223 Myofibroblasts differentiation: Microphotography of coal workers' pneumoconiosis showing pulmonary interstitial fibrosis, evidenced by the dense collagen stained with pink shown in A (H.E stain) or blue shown in B (Masson stain). C AND D (regional amplification of C), Immunoreactivity for α-smooth muscle actin confirms the spindle or polygonal cells in the nodules are myofibroblasts. (From the patient, working in rock drilling for 22 years)

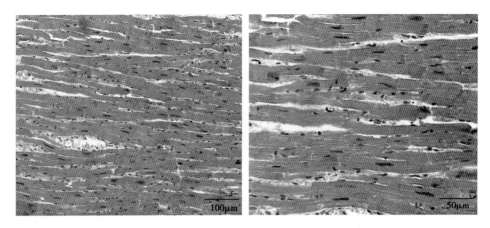

图224　正常心肌组织(右心室):心肌纤维(细胞)排列整齐,心肌纤维间有少量结缔组织。(H.E染色)

Fig.224　Normal heart tissue (from right ventricle): The myocytes arranges in a linear fashion orderly, with minimal connective tissue between cells. (H.E stain)

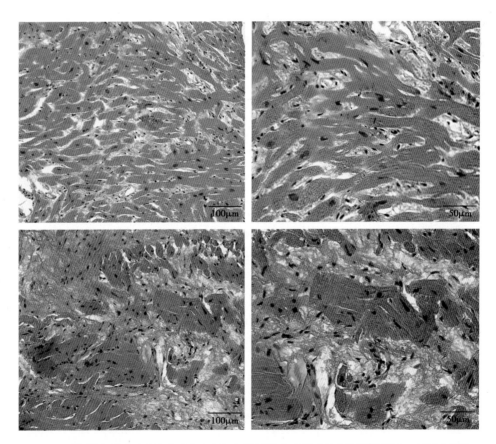

图225　肺源性心脏病心肌组织(右心室):心肌纤维瘢痕形成伴心肌细胞肥大。(井下采煤工作18年,煤场放煤工作10年)(H.E染色)

Fig.225　Right ventricle with cor pulmonale: High power view of right ventricle illustrates the details of scar tissue and myocyte with hypertrophy. (From the patient, working coal mining and issuing for 18 years and 10 years respectively) (H.E stain)

第三部分
煤工尘肺案例

Part III
Cases of Coal Workers' Pneumoconiosis

案例一

煤矽肺I期(结节 + 尘斑 - 气肿)

职业史

男性,65岁,井下采煤及掘进工作17年。

临床情况

1963年3月,因患有肺结核病转入劳保待遇,于1965年退休。1978年12月26日,因心肺功能不好,住院观察、治疗。病情严重,治疗无效而死亡。

肺部尸检情况

大体检查:两肺内黑色结节状病灶达30个。肺内诸多煤斑灶伴肺气肿形成,肺间质纤维化较明显。肺门、气管叉及气管旁淋巴结内可见多数黑色结节,并融合成块,最大达1.5cm。两肺尖部胸膜粘连、纤维性增厚。

显微镜检查:两肺内有诸多煤尘细胞性结节及少量煤矽结节形成伴小叶中心型肺气肿。同时可见煤斑及煤尘灶形成。肺间质纤维化明显。胸膜局部煤尘大量沉积伴纤维组织及小血管增生,局部增厚的胸膜形成城垛样结构。肺内局部区域伴有化脓性炎症与浆液渗出性炎症。

病理诊断:

1. 煤矽肺I期 细胞性结节及煤矽结节总数达30个,伴明显的间质纤维化。
2. 肺门、支气管叉和气管旁淋巴结内煤矽结节形成并融合。
3. 化脓性支气管肺炎。
4. 胸膜粘连、纤维性增厚。

Case 1

Anthracosilicosis
(stage I, Nodules and maculae surrounded by emphysema)

Age: 65 years

Sex: Male

Occupational History:

The patient had been performed coal mining and tunneling for 17 years.

Medical History:

The patient was diagnosed with pulmonary tuberculosis in March, 1963 and retired in 1965. On December 26, 1978, he was attained to hospital with pulmonary and cardiac malaise. Although having treatment, his symptoms were more and more severe, and finally death.

Autopsy examination of the lung:

Gross: The lungs were stunned with close to thirty of black nodules and abundant coal dust maculae surrounded by emphysema, as well as obvious interstitial fibrosis. The black nodules in the lymph nodes of hilum, bifurcation of tracheas, para tracheas were partially merged, forming some massive lesions with 1.5cm in maximum diameter. In addition, pleural adhesion and fibrous thickening are visible in the tips of the lungs.

Histology: The microscopic view of the lungs shows abundant cellular coal dust nodules and obvious interstitial fibrosis, with a few amount of coal silicotic nodules surrounded by centriacinar emphysema, coal dust dots, and coal dust foci. A patchy of thickening pleura contained coal dusts deposits, proliferated collagen fibers and small blood vessels, resembling "city battlements". Regional airspace filled with neutrophils infiltration and serous exudation response to suppurative inflammation and exudative inflammation.

Pathological Diagnosis:

1. Anthracosilicosis (stage I): It is supported by close to thirty of cellular nodules and coal silicotic nodules as well as obvious interstitial fibrosis.

2. Coalescence of coal silicotic nodules in the lymph nodes of hilum, bifurcation of tracheas, para tracheas.

3. Suppurative bronchopneumonia.

4. Pleural adhesion and fibrous thickening.

案例一　附图（Appendix of case 1）

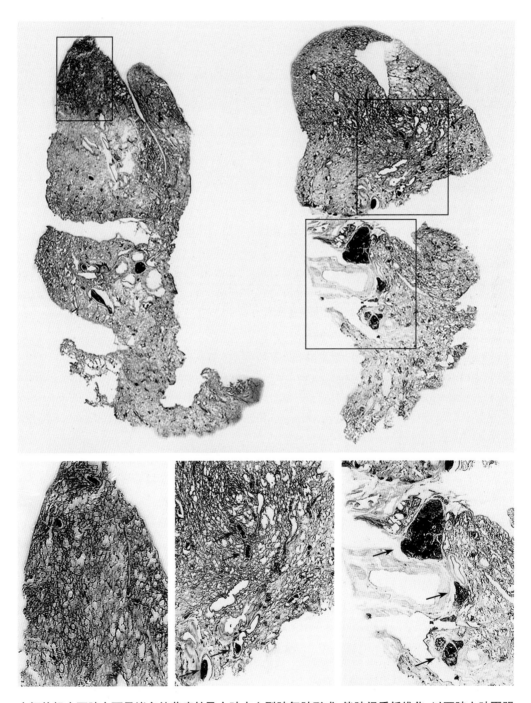

大切片标本两肺内可见诸多结节病灶及小叶中心型肺气肿形成，伴肺间质纤维化，以两肺上叶更明显。肺门淋巴结肿大（红色箭头所指为结节病灶，黑色箭头为肿大的肺门淋巴结）。

Large slice of lungs illustration of moderate amount of nodular lesions (red arrows) and centriacinar emphysema as well as interstitial fibrosis, which are more severe in the upper lobes. Note the enlarged hilar lymph nodes (black arrows).

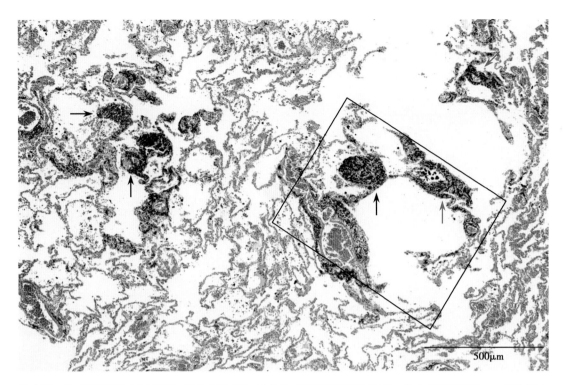

肺内煤尘沉积形成煤尘细胞灶和煤尘细胞性结节病变,伴灶旁肺气肿形成。肺小血管扩张充血,肺泡腔内炎细胞渗出(红色箭头指煤尘细胞灶,黑色箭头指煤尘细胞性结节)。(H.E 染色)

Coal dust causes cellular coal dust foci (red arrows) and cellular coal dust nodules (black arrows), surrounded by emphysema. The congested small blood vessels are associated with inflammatory cells infiltration in the airspace. (H.E stain)

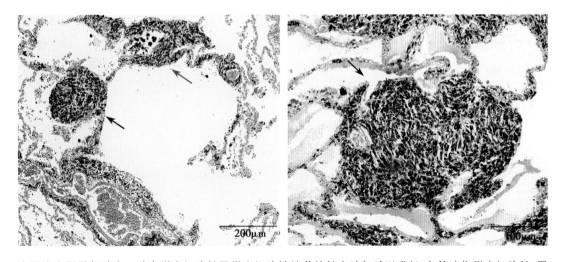

左图为上图局部放大。肺内煤尘细胞灶及煤尘细胞性结节伴灶旁肺气肿形成(红色箭头指煤尘细胞灶,黑色箭头指煤尘细胞性结节。(H.E 染色)

Left photography, showing the details of above, evidence of cellular coal dust foci (red arrow) and cellular coal dust nodules (black arrow), which are surrounded by emphysema. (H.E stain)

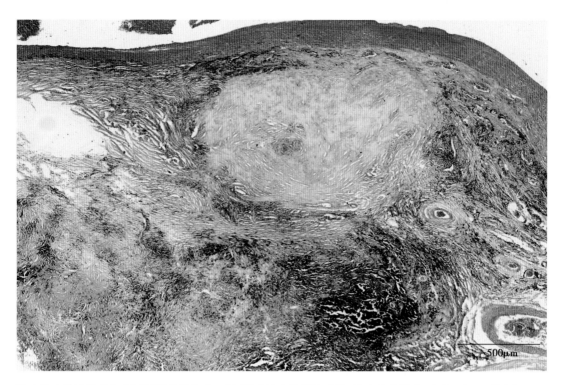

肺内较大的矽结节与间质纤维化融合在一起,形成较大的团块病灶,伴小血管增生、充血。(H.E 染色)

A larger silicotic nodule and the surrounding interstitial fibrous tissue undergo coalescence process, forming a much bigger lesion. Note small blood vessels hyperplasia and congestion. (H.E stain)

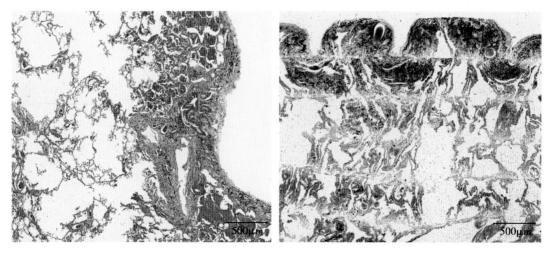

胸膜内较多煤尘沉积,伴纤维组织增生,胸膜纤维性增厚。胸膜内及胸膜直下小血管增生、充血。胸膜下肺组织间质纤维化。(H.E 染色)

The thickening pleura contains coal dusts deposits, proliferated collagen fibers and small blood vessels, the tissue under the pleura reveals interstitial fibrosis and small vessel hyperplasia, congestion. (H.E stain)

案例二

煤肺I期(煤尘斑灶 + 细胞性结节)

职业史

男性,40 岁,井下掘进工作 8 年,回采煤工作 7 年。

临床情况

房室传导阻滞伴心衰 5 年余。此次因病情加重住院,于 1979 年 11 月 27 日抢救无效死亡。

临床诊断:完全性房室传导阻、心衰。

肺部尸检情况

大体检查:胸膜煤斑灶弥漫分布,但数量不多(直径在 0.1~0.3cm)。肺内煤斑灶散在分布,可见数多境界较清晰黑色小结节,全肺超过 20 个。伴轻度肺气肿和肺间质纤维化形成,肺门淋巴结略有肿大(见图谱中图 7、图 8)。

显微镜检查:两肺内有诸多煤尘细胞灶及煤尘纤维灶形成伴小叶中心型肺气肿。可见较多细胞性结节(煤尘细胞性结节/煤尘细胞纤维性结节)形成。未见矽结节或煤矽结节形成。肺间质轻度纤维化。

病理诊断:

1. 煤肺I期　细胞性结节(煤尘细胞性结节/煤尘细胞纤维性结节)超过 20 个,伴轻度间质纤维化与轻度肺气肿形成。

2. 肺门淋巴结内煤尘沉积伴尘性纤维化。

注:①此病例肺组织是以煤尘斑灶(煤尘细胞灶/煤尘纤维灶)与细胞性结节(煤尘细胞性结节/煤尘细胞纤维性结节)形成为主要病变特点,在肺内与肺门淋巴结内均没有查找到典型的矽结节和煤矽结节的形成。可作为煤肺一个病例的诊断。②从病理形态学变化观察可见,病变有一个由巨噬细胞性肺泡炎——煤尘细胞性结节——煤尘细胞纤维性结节逐步演变与形成的过程。这可能也是煤肺病变形成的特点之一。

Case 2

Anthracosis
(stage I, Coal dust maculae and cellular nodules)

Age: 40 years

Sex: Male

Occupational History:

The patient had been performed coal tunneling and mining for 8 years and 7 years respectively.

Medical History:

The patient had five years of atrioventricular block and heart failure, and went to hospital because of more and more severe symptoms, On November 27, 1979, after the rescue battlement, he unfortunately died from complete atrioventricular block and heart failure.

Autopsy examination of the lung:

Gross: Minimal coal dust maculae are widely distributed in pleura, which diameters range from 0.1cm to 0.3cm. Scattered coal dust maculae in lung show a well-demarcated, small, black nodular appearance, totally more than twenty in quantity. Mild emphysema and interstitial fibrosis as well as enlarged hilar lymph nodes could be seen (Fig. 7 and 8).

Histology: The lungs are characterized by cellular coal dust foci and fibrous coal dust foci surrounded by centriacinar emphysema. The nodular lesions, such as cellular coal dust nodules and cellular fibrous coal dust nodules, are present in lung, but no silicotic nodules or coal silicotic nodules. Note mild proliferation of fibrous tissue in the interstitial tissue.

Pathological Diagnosis:

1. Anthracosis (stage I): it is supported by over twenty of cellular nodules (cellular coal dust nodules and cellular fibrous coal dust nodules) and mild emphysema and interstitial fibrosis.

2. Hilar lymph nodes fibrosis with coal dust deposition.

Comments:

1) The distinctive feature of this case is the formation of coal dust foci (cellular foci and fibrous foci) and coal dust nodules (cellular nodules and cellular fibrous nodules), without typical silicotic nodules and coal silicotic nodules in both pulmonary tissue and hilar lymph nodes, supporting the diagnosis with anthracosis.

2) Morphology of this case provides evidence of the disease development in the order of macrophage alveolitis, cellular coal dust nodules, and cellular fibrous coal dust nodules, which may be referred as a characteristic of anthracosis.

案例二 附图(Appendix of case 2)

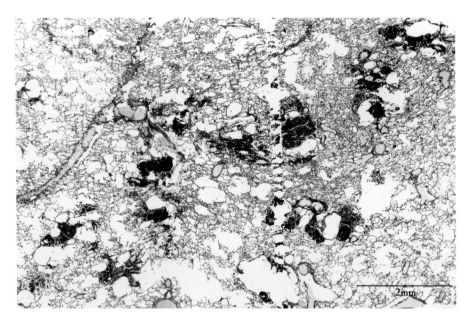

肺内诸多煤尘细胞灶及煤尘细胞性结节形成,伴轻度灶旁肺气肿形成。(H.E 染色)
Moderate amount of cellular coal dust foci and cellular coal dust nodules are accompanied by mild emphysema close to the lesions. (H.E stain)

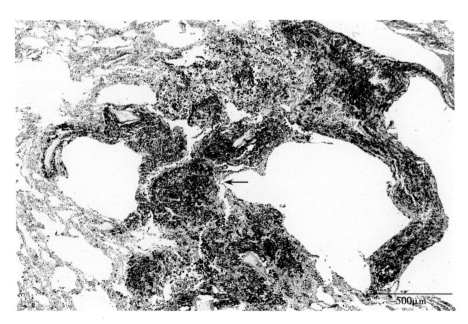

肺内诸多煤尘细胞灶及煤尘细胞性结节形成(箭头所指),伴轻度灶旁肺气肿形成。(H.E 染色)
Moderate amount of cellular coal dust foci and cellular coal dust nodules (arrow) are accompanied by mild emphysema close to the lesions. (H.E stain)

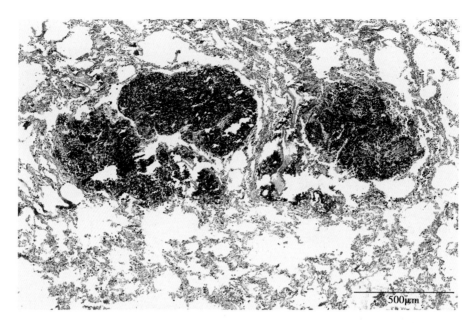

肺内煤尘细胞性结节形成,伴轻度灶旁肺气肿形成。(H.E 染色)
Cellular coal dust nodules are accompanied by mild emphysema close to the lesions in lung. (H.E stain)

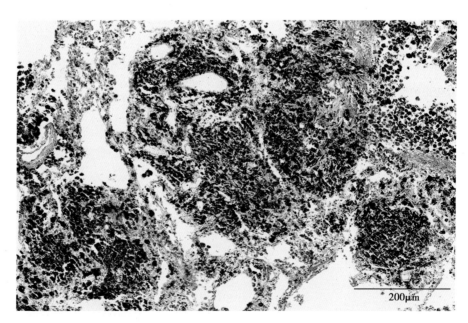

肺内煤尘细胞性结节形成。(H.E 染色)
Cellular coal dust nodules in lung. (H.E stain)

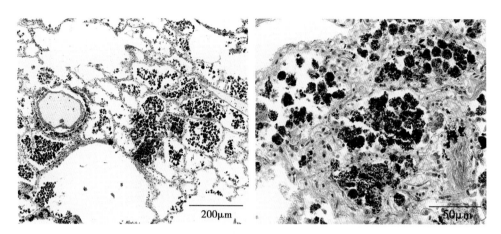

巨噬细胞性肺泡炎。(H.E 染色)
Macrophage alveolitis in lung. (H.E stain)

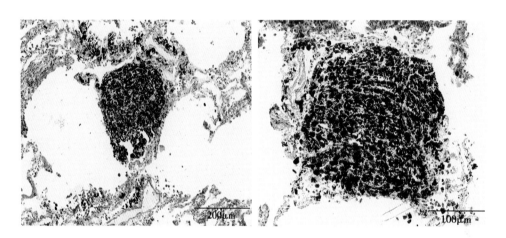

肺内煤尘细胞性结节。(H.E 染色)
Cellular coal dust nodules in lung. (H.E stain)

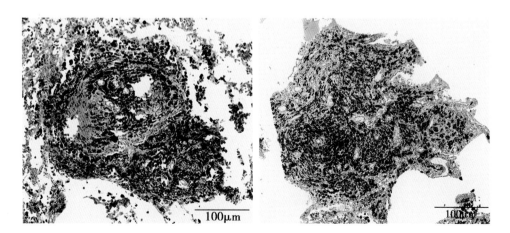

肺内煤尘细胞纤维性结节。(H.E 染色)
Cellular fibrous coal dust nodules in lung. (H.E stain)

案例三

煤矽肺Ⅱ期(尘斑－气肿型)

职业史

男性,57 岁,井下掘进工作 26 年,井下看运煤传送带 12 年。

临床情况

慢性支气管炎、肺气肿病史 19 年。其间多次住院治疗。此次于 1985 年 12 月 7 日因肺部感染、呼吸困难而入院。查体:桶状胸,肋间隙增宽。双肺叩诊过浊音、听诊双肺湿性啰音。X 线胸片透光度增高,纹理增多、增粗。双肺中下外侧带可见纤细的编织网状影。双肺门阴影增大。于 1985 年 12 月 9 日医治无效死亡。

临床诊断为肺气肿合并感染、肺心病、呼吸衰竭。

肺部尸检情况

大体检查:双肺胸膜粘连增厚,以中下 2/3 区域严重。双肺上叶肺大疱明显。双肺灰黑色,煤斑灶密集,局部融合成片伴小叶中心型肺气肿,占双肺容(面)积的 75%(见图谱中图 1)。

显微镜检查:两肺诸多煤斑、煤尘纤维灶伴肺气肿。大泡型肺气肿形成。肺弥漫性间质纤维化达到 2 级 /2 度。肺水肿。支气管慢性炎症。肺门、支气管叉和气管旁淋巴结内尘性纤维化。

病理诊断:

1. 煤矽肺Ⅱ期(尘斑-气肿型)　尘斑-气肿占肺容(面)积 75%,弥漫性间质纤维化达到 2 级 /2 度。

2. 肺内多个肺大疱形成。

3. 肺门、支气管叉和气管旁淋巴结内尘性纤维化。

4. 慢性支气管炎。

5. 胸膜粘连增厚。

Case 3

Anthracosilicosis
(stage II, Coal dust maculae and emphysema)

Age: 57 years

Sex: Male

Occupational History:

The patient had been performed coal tunneling for 26 years and coal transportation for 12 years.

Medical History:

Nineteen years of chronic bronchitis and emphysema with occasional clinical treatment. On December 7, 1985, the patient suffered pulmonary infection and dyspnea, being in hospital. Physical examination found barrel chest and widened intercostals space. Dullness and wet rale of lungs were easily captured. X-ray revealed an increased lucent lung with increased lung marking, delicate interwoven image in lateral parts of middle lobe and lower lobes, as well as enlarged hilar shadow of the lungs. On December 9, 1985, after the rescue battlement, he unfortunately died from emphysema with pulmonary infection, pulmonary heart disease and respiratory failure.

Autopsy examination of the lung:

Gross: Pleura of both lungs become thickening and adhesion, which is more severe in the lower and middle third of the pleura. The black-gray lungs are riddled with coal dust maculae, some of which getting fusion, surrounded by extensive area of centriacinar emphysema (the area of emphysema is 75% of the whole lungs). In the upper lobes of both lungs, bullae are clearly seen. (Fig. 1)

Histology: Moderate amount of coal dust dots and fibrous coal dust foci are widely distributed in lungs with bullous emphysema, diffuse interstitial fibrosis (grade II), pneumonedema and chronic bronchitis. Fibrous proliferation, mixed with coal dust deposits, is present in the lymph nodes of hilum, bifurcation of tracheas, para tracheas.

Pathological Diagnosis:

1. Anthracosilicosis (stage II, type of coal dust dot-emphysema): It is supported by extensive area of coal dust dots and emphysema (the area of lesions occupied 75% of the whole lung) and diffuse interstitial fibrosis (grade II).

2. Bullous emphysema.

3. Fibrous proliferation with coal dust deposition in the lymph nodes of hilum, bifurcation of tracheas, para tracheas.

4. Chronic bronchitis.

5. Pleural adhesion and thickening.

案例三　附图（Appendix of case 3）

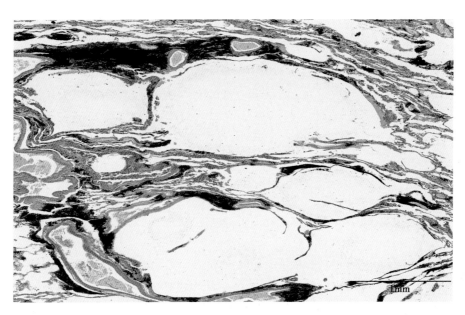

煤尘沉积在终末细支气管、呼吸性细支气管及肺泡壁和小血管周围，小气道明显扩张，形成"尘斑 - 气肿"病变，伴间质纤维化。（H.E 染色）

Coal dust deposited around terminal bronchia, respiratory bronchia, alveolar septum and small blood vessels is admixed with enlarged small airway, producing the lesion of "coal dust dots-emphysema". Interstitial fibrosis is visible. (H.E stain)

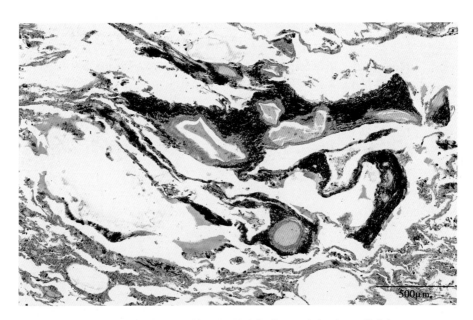

煤尘沉积在呼吸性细支气管及小血管周围，伴小气道明显扩张。（H.E 染色）

Minimal coal dust deposition around respiratory bronchia and small blood vessels, with enlarged small airway. (H.E stain)

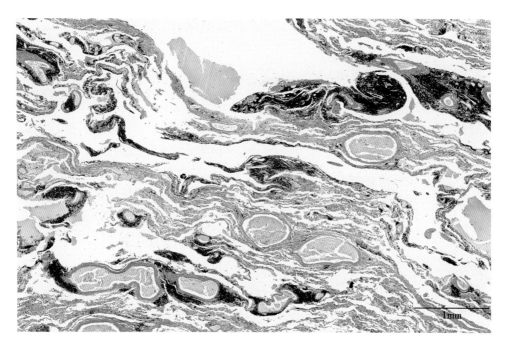

煤尘沉积在终末小气道和小血管周围,小气道扩张,伴明显的间质纤维化。(H.E 染色)
Minimal coal dust deposition around terminal bronchia and small blood vessels, with enlarged small airway and obvious interstitial fibrosis. (H.E stain)

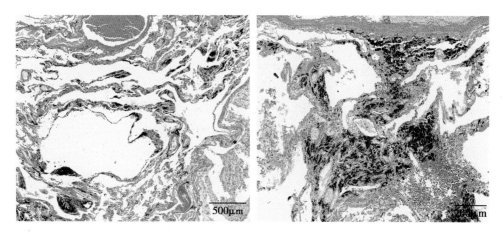

左图显示"尘斑 - 气肿"病变伴弥漫性间质纤维化;右图显示弥漫性间质纤维化。(H.E 染色)
The left photography illustration of "coal dust dots and emphysema"and diffuse interstitial fibrosis; while the right one evidence of diffuse interstitial fibrosis. (H.E stain)

案例四

煤矽肺Ⅲ期(大块纤维化)

职业史

男性,77 岁,井下凿岩工作 32 年。

临床情况

慢性支气管炎 10 余年,日渐加重。每年均因咳喘住院治疗。诊断为慢性阻塞性肺病,肺心病,冠心病,曾有肺结核病史。

1985 年 8 月 15 日因咳嗽、气喘加重伴心慌住院。

X 线胸片检查发现,两肺上叶外侧均有 5.0×4.0cm 对称块状阴影,内有透亮区。两肺底部和肺尖部有肺大疱。

入院诊断为慢性支气管炎,肺气肿,肺感染,冠心病伴心衰。

入院后对症治疗,病情不见好转,于 1985 年 8 月 30 日上午 12 时死亡。

肺部尸检情况

大体检查: 两肺上叶可见大块状纤维化区域(左肺 8.5cm×6.5cm,右肺 8.0cm×7.0cm),其内有空洞形成,含较多坏死性物质。两肺重度弥漫性间质纤维化,以两肺上叶接近块状纤维化区域更为明显,局部纤维化区域呈"垂柳状"外观。两肺肺内弥漫性煤尘斑灶及灶周肺气肿形成。弥漫性囊泡型肺气肿及大泡型肺气肿形成。局部支气管壁增厚、扩张。胸膜肥厚,灰白硬韧,有明显的纤维性粘连,以两肺上叶最为显著(见图谱中图 19- 图 22)。

显微镜检查: 两肺可见诸多煤尘斑、煤尘纤维灶和较多煤矽结节。除块状纤维化区域大量胶原纤维沉积外,肺弥漫性间质纤维化明显。肺门淋巴结内煤尘沉积,煤矽结节及煤矽结核结节形成。肺内支气管壁炎细胞浸润,管壁纤维化,管腔内可见较多见炎性渗出物。慢性炎性空洞形成,空洞壁炎性纤维组织增生。

病理诊断:

1. 煤矽肺Ⅲ期   两肺上叶大块纤维化伴空洞形成,肺内重度弥漫性间质纤维化。
2. 肺内弥漫性煤尘灶及灶周肺气肿形成。肺内弥漫性囊泡型肺气肿及大泡型肺气肿形成。
3. 肺门、气管叉、气管旁淋巴结内多数煤矽结节形成并融合、硬化伴有钙化。
4. 胸膜肥厚,纤维性粘连,以两肺上叶为显著。
5. 慢性支气管炎及支气管扩张。

Case 4
Anthracosilicosis
(stage III, Massive fibrosis)

Age: 77 years

Sex: Male

Occupational History:

The patient had been performed rock drilling for 32 years.

Medical History:

More than ten years of chronic bronchitis and tuberculosis, clinical treatment failing in prohibiting the disease development, finally advancing chronic obstructive pulmonary disease, pulmonary heart disease and coronary heart disease. On August 15,1985, the patient was flustered and felt his serious cough and asthma. X-ray revealed the bilaterally symmetrical lucent images with extensive area of 5.0cm*4.0cm in the upper lobes, and several bullae in the tips and bottom of lungs. He was diagnosed with chronic bronchitis, pulmonary emphysema, pulmonary infection, coronary heart disease with heart failure, and was in hospital. After having treatment, his symptoms were kept. He unfortunately died on 12 a.m, August 30,1985.

Autopsy examination of the lung:

Gross: Gross view of the upper lobes reveals the irregular cavities lined by caseous materials, entrapped in the massive fibrotic lesions (the area in left lung is 8.5cm*6.5cm, the one in right lung is 8.0cm*7.0cm). The fibrous proliferation in the interstitial tissue is so severe that it is widely distributed in both lungs, especially in the upper lobes, adjacent to the lesions of massive fibrosis. Drooping willows of the proliferated fibrous tissue could be seen. Both of lungs are stunned with coal dust foci surrounded by emphysema, with scattered cystic emphysema and bullous emphysema. A segment of the enlarged bronchi shows a thickening wall. The gray-white pleura is the consequence of thickening response and adhesion, which is most obvious in the upper lobes.(Fig. 19-Fig. 22)

Histology: Microscopic photography evidence of moderate amount of coal dust dots, fibrous coal dust foci and coal silicotic nodules, with abundant proliferated fibrous tissue in the lesions of massive fibrosis and in the interstitial tissue. Coal silicotic nodules and coal silicotic tuberculous nodules are also visible in the coal dust-deposited hilar lymph nodes. Inflammatory cells infiltrate in fibrous bronchial wall with inflammatory exudation in lumen, and meanwhile inflammation evacuates the inflammatory debris, creating a cavity lined by fibrous tissue.

Pathological diagnosis:

1. Anthracosilicosis (stage Ⅲ): It is supported by upper lobes of massive fibrosis and multiple areas of cavitation, as well as severe diffuse interstitial fibrosis.

2. Scattered coal dust foci surrounded by emphysema, with distributed cystic emphysema and bullous emphysema.

3. Multiple coal silicotic nodules in the lymph nodes of hilum, bifurcation of tracheas, para tracheas, some of which undergoing the changes of coalescence, sclerosis and calcification.

4. Pleural adhesion and thickening, especially in the upper parts.

5. Chronic bronchitis and bronchiectasis.

案例四 附图(Appendix of case 4)

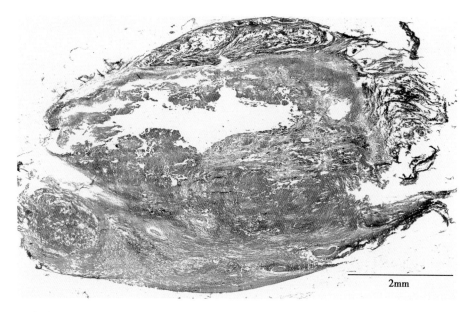

2mm

融合性矽结节与增生的纤维组织混合在一起构成纤维性巨块状病变,其间可见较多煤尘沉积。(H.E 染色)

A fibrous massive lesion, composed by confluent silicotic nodules and proliferated fibrous tissue, is studded with coal dusts deposition. (H.E stain)

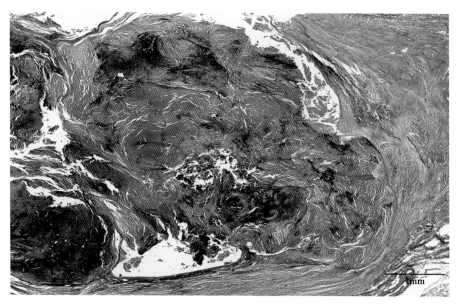

1mm

融合性矽结节与增生的纤维组织混合在一起构成纤维性巨块状病变,大量煤尘沉积在块状纤维化区域内。(H.E 染色)

A fibrous massive lesion is admixture of fused silicotic nodules and proliferated fibrous tissue, with ornament of abundant coal dust deposits. (H.E stain)

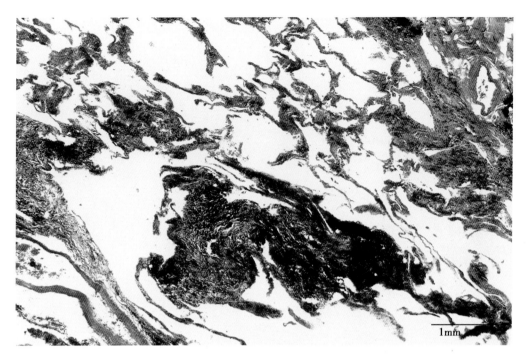

煤尘纤维灶形成：肺内煤尘纤维灶形成伴弥漫性间质纤维化。(H.E 染色)

Fibrous coal dust foci: Fibrous coal dust foci are accompanied by diffuse interstitial fibrosis in lung. (H.E stain)

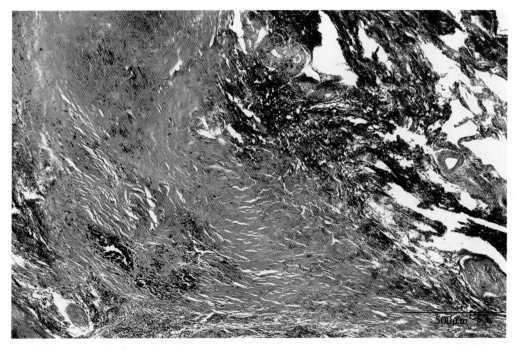

块状纤维化空洞形成：空洞壁为增生的纤维组织与沉积的煤尘及部分变性坏死组织构成。(H.E 染色)

Massive fibrosis with cavitation. The cavity entrapped in the massive fibrosis is lined by proliferated fibrous tissue, coal dust deposits, and tissue debris. (H.E stain)

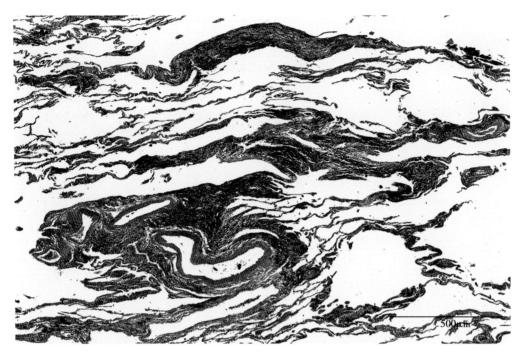

煤尘沉积与弥漫增生的纤维组织混杂在一起，伴小气道的扩张。（H.E 染色）
Microscopic view of lung shows the mixture of coal dust and diffusely scattered fibrous tissue, accompanied by small airway expansion. (H.E stain)

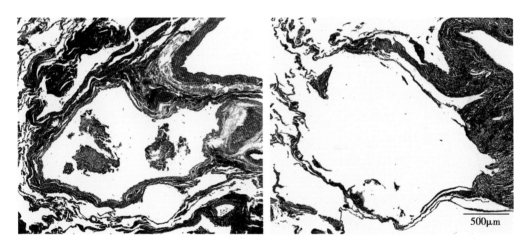

左图为尘性细支气管炎伴间质纤维化。煤尘沉积在细气管壁伴纤维组织增生，细支气管上皮细胞脱落与粘液样坏死物混杂形成粘液栓。细支气管周围间质纤维化明显。右图为呼吸性细支气管扩张。煤尘沉积在呼吸性细气管管壁伴纤维组织增生，管壁增厚，管腔扩张。（H.E 染色）
(Left) Coal bronchiolitis with interstitial fibrosis. Coal dust deposits in bronchiole wall, and a mucous plug containing exfoliated epithelial cells and mucoid tissue debris in lumen. Fibrous proliferation occurs in bronchiole wall or close to the bronchioles. (Right) Respiratory bronchioles dilation. In coal dust-deposited respiratory bronchioles, its lumen becomes larger and the wall is thickening due to fibrous proliferation tissue. (H.E stain)

案例五

煤矽肺Ⅲ期合并肺结核病

职业史

男性,42岁,井下机电维修工作20年。

临床情况

1980年初,因发烧胸痛就诊,当时疑似肺结核门诊抗结核治疗。后X线胸片发现左肺近肺门部有一直径3cm大小的肿物,考虑中心型肺癌,经用钴^{60}放射治疗一个疗程,病情略有好转。于1981年3月再次出现高烧不退、胸痛,气短。X线检查左肺肿物渐大,肺上叶片状阴影。抗炎对症治疗无效,于1981年3月24日因呼吸衰竭死亡。

肺部尸检情况

大体检查:左肺上叶灰白色、弥漫实变,近肺门部有一4.0cm×3.0cm形状不规则的空洞。左肺上叶下部、下叶上部近肺门处有一3.5cm×3.0cm黑色实变区域,质地硬韧,其间有数个点状白色病灶。右肺全肺散在粟粒大小白色实性灶。黑色斑灶病变散在分布左、右两肺(见图谱中图31、图32)。

显微镜检查:两肺可见诸多煤尘斑、煤尘纤维灶和较多煤矽结核结节。干酪样坏死性结核病灶遍布肺内。除块状纤维化区域大量胶原纤维沉积外,肺弥漫性间质纤维化较明显。肺门淋巴结内煤尘沉积,煤矽结及煤矽结核结节形成。

病理诊断:

1. 煤矽肺Ⅲ期　左肺上叶下部及下叶上部块状纤维化形成。
2. (左肺上叶)大叶性干酪性肺炎及空洞形成。
3. 肺(播散性)粟粒性肺结核。
4. 肺门及气管叉淋巴结内多数煤矽结节及煤矽结核结节形成。

Case 5

Anthracosilicosis
(stage III) with pulmonary tuberculosis

Age: 42 years

Sex: Male

Occupational History:

The patient had been performed underground maintenance of equipment and electricity for 20 years.

Medical History:

Since the beginning of 1980, the patient had been in fever and chest pain, being diagnosed with pulmonary tuberculosis and receiving anti-tuberculosis therapy. Then, he was found with central lung cancer, evidenced by a, adjacent to hilum, 3cm in diameter, mass in the left lung by X-ray, and received a course of cobalt-60 radiotherapy which temporarily ameliorated his symptom. On March, 1981, however, he had high fever and felt chest pain as well as shortness of breath again, with X-ray examination of enlarging mass and patchy shadows of upper lobes. After anti-inflammatory therapy, his symptoms were kept and died from respiratory failure on March 24, 1981.

Autopsy examination of the lung:

Gross: In the diffusely consolidated, gray-white upper lobes of the left lung, a 4.0cm*3.0cm area of irregular cavity is close to the hilum, and a consolidated, 3.5cm*3.0cm in area, black, firm lesion, containing several white tuberculosis sites, emerges in the airspace of the lower part of the upper lobe or the upper part of the lower lobe, adjacent to the hilum. Miliary tuberculosis, showing multiple consolidated gray-white lesions, is widely distributed in the right lung. The scattered black coal dust maculae are clearly visible in lungs. (Fig.31, Fig.32)

Histology: Multiple coal dust dots, fibrous coal dust foci, and coal silicotic tuberculous nodules could be seen in both of lungs decorated with distributed caseous necrosis. Abundant proliferated fibrous tissue deposits in the lesions of massive fibrosis and in the interstitial tissue. Coal silicotic nodules and coal silicotic tuberculous nodules are also visible in the coal dust-deposited hilar lymph nodes.

Pathological diagnosis:

1. Anthracosilicosis (stage III): It is supported by the obvious massive fibrous which locates at the lower part of upper lobe or upper part of lower lobe, in the left lung.

2. Caseous lobar pneumonia with cavities in upper lobe of the left lung.

3. Disseminated miliary tuberculosis in lung.

4. Coal silicotic nodules and coal silicotic tuberculous nodules in the lymph nodes of hilum and bifurcation of tracheas.

案例五　附图（Appendix of case 5）

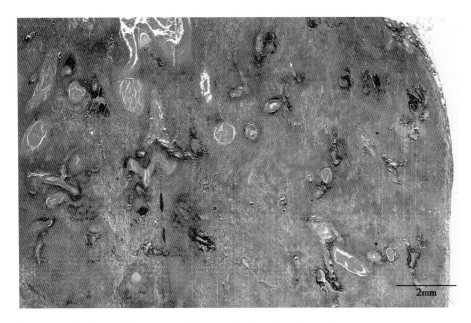

增生的纤维组织团块中尚可见煤尘沉积形成的煤尘斑灶病变、坏死性结节状病变及增生小血管的轮廓。（H.E 染色）

The outline of coal dust maculae, necrotic nodules and proliferated small blood vessels may still be recognized in the proliferated fibrous mass. (H.E stain)

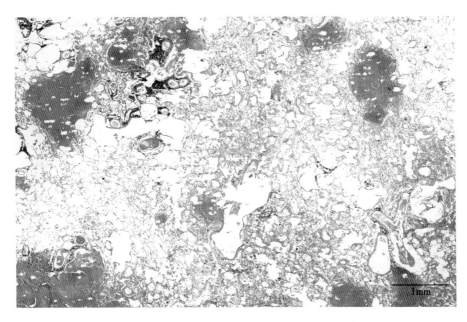

肺内可见"尘斑 - 气肿"和多个干酪样坏死实变病灶。（H.E 染色）

Coal dust dots-emphysemas in lung are accompanied by multiple consolodated caseous lesions. (H.E stain)

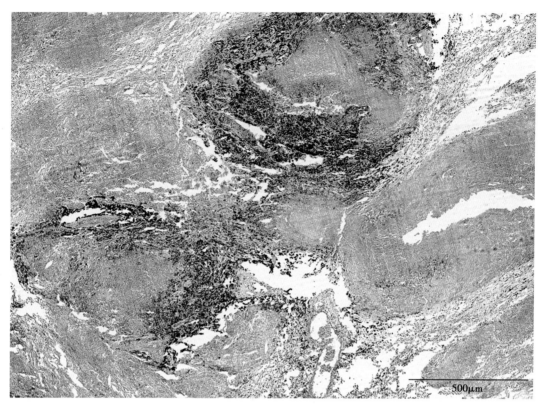

肺内煤矽结核结节形成,周围肺泡腔内充填着干酪样坏死与炎性渗出。(H.E 染色)
Microscopic view illustration of coal silicotic tuberculous nodules, surrounded by caseous necrosis and inflammatory exudates filling in the airspaces. (H.E stain)

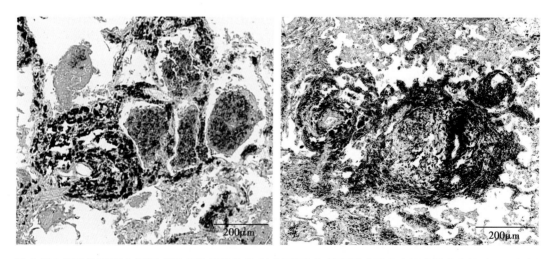

肺内煤尘细胞性结节(左图)和煤尘细胞纤维性结节(右图)形成,周围肺泡腔内充填炎性渗出物。(H.E 染色)
Photography of lung illustration of the formation of cellular coal dust nodules (left) and cellular fibrous coal dust nodules (right), accompanied by inflammatory exudates filling in the surrounding airspace. (H.E stain)

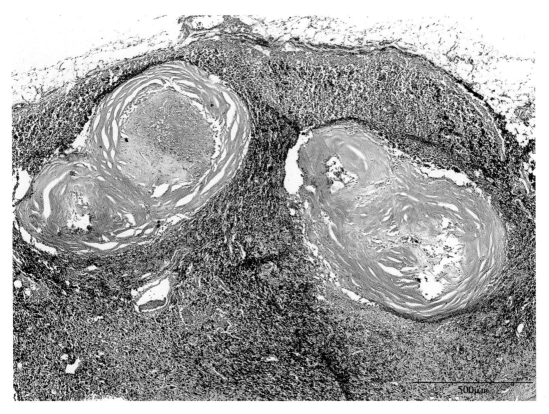

大量煤尘沉积在淋巴结内，可见两个煤矽结核结节形成。(H.E 染色)

Two coal silicotic tuberculous nodules emerge in the coal dust-deposited lymph node. (H.E stain)

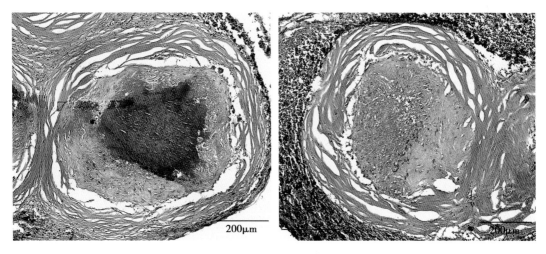

淋巴结内煤矽结核结节形成。(H.E 染色)

High power view of lymph node shows the details of coal silicotic tuberculous nodules. (H.E stain)

案例六

煤矽肺Ⅲ期合并肺癌

职业史

男性,52 岁,井下掘进工作 5 年,井下采煤工作 20 年。

临床情况

于 1984 年 6 月普查时发现右肺上叶密度增高阴影。咳嗽、咳痰,呼吸困难加重一个月。入院后病情逐渐加重,恶病质体质,双肺遍布水泡音。X 线胸片双肺为云絮状密度增高阴影。白细胞计数增高。经消炎、对症、支持疗法等治疗后病情不见好转,且逐日恶化,呼吸困难加重。痰中查到可疑癌细胞。于 1984 年 10 月 5 日,因呼吸功能与心脏功能衰竭而死亡。

临床诊断:晚期肺癌。

肺部尸检情况

大体检查:右肺上叶下部有一 6.0cm×5.0cm×5.0cm 块状纤维化病变。近叶间裂胸膜处有一裂隙样空洞,腔内储满墨汁样坏死物。大块纤维化相应侧面胸膜呈不整形疤痕收缩性凹陷。肺内大量煤斑灶及小叶中心型肺气肿形成。弥漫性灰白色结节样肿块分布全肺(见图谱中图 40)。

显微镜检查:两肺诸多煤斑、煤尘纤维灶伴小叶中心型肺气肿。偶见非典型煤矽结节形成。肺内重度弥漫性间质纤维化,胸膜增厚、纤维化显著。肺内可见诸多腺泡样癌巢,浸润性生长,破坏原有肺组织结构。肺内合并感染。肺门淋巴结矽结节形成及尘性纤维化。支气管叉、支气管旁淋巴结均有癌转移。

病理诊断:

1. 煤矽肺Ⅲ期　进行性块状纤维化形成。
2. 肺内大量煤斑灶伴小叶中心型肺气肿,肺重度尘性间质纤维化。
3. 肺门淋巴结内煤矽结节形成及尘性纤维化。
4. 支气管炎、支气管肺炎。
5. 胸膜增厚、纤维化。
6. 肺癌(腺癌)。

Case 6

Anthracosilicosis
(stage III) with lung cancer

Age: 52 years

Sex: Male

Occupational History:

The patient had been performed coal tunneling and mining for 5 years and 20 years respectively.

Medical History:

In June, 1984, health examination found a high density shade in the upper lobe of the right lung. For one month that followed, the patient had complained the more and more severe symptoms of cough, hemoptysis, aspiration difficulty, and then was attained to hospital. After examination, cachexia was shown clearly, the rale was widely heard in lung, and leukocytes increased. X-ray of lung revealed the cloudy, high density shades. The treatment of inhibiting inflammation response, relieving some of the symptoms and nutrition had no benefits on him, and he took a turn for the worse. Suspicious cancer cells were positively found in his phlegm. On October 5, 1984, he unfortunately died from the respiratory failure and heart failure.

Clinical diagnosis: Advanced lung cancer.

Autopsy examination of the lung:

Gross: In the right lung, the massive fibrosis, 6.0cm*5.0cm*5.0cm in size, emerges in the lower part of the upper lobe, above which the pleura with an irregular scar tissue is refracted; and a slit-shaped cavity that are full of black tissue debris is adjacent to the interlobar fissure. The whole lungs are riddled with coal dust maculae surrounded by centriacinar emphysema, interspersed with gray-white nodular masses. (Fig. 40)

Histology: abundant coal dust dots and fibrous coal dust foci surrounded by centriacinar emphysema are scattered in the whole lungs, with occasional atypical coal silicotic nodules and severe interstitial fibrosis as well as thickening pleura. Meanwhile, the invasion of glandular cancer nests destructs the pulmonary tissue, inducing inflammatory response. Silicotic nodules are visible in the hilar lymph nodes with coal dust-deposited fibrous tissue. Adenocarcinoma metastasis occurs in the lymph nodes of bifurcation of tracheas and para tracheas.

Pathological diagnosis:

1. Anthracosilicosis (stage III): It is supported by the obvious massive fibrousin the lungs.

2. Abundant coal dust maculae surrounded by centriacinar emphysema, and severe interstitial fibrosis with coal dust deposition.

3. Coal silicotic nodules in the hilar lymph nodes with coal dust-deposited fibrous tissue.

4. Bronchitis and bronchopneumonia.

5. Pleural thickening and fibrousis.

6. Pulmonary adenocarcinoma.

案例六　附图（Appendix of case 6）

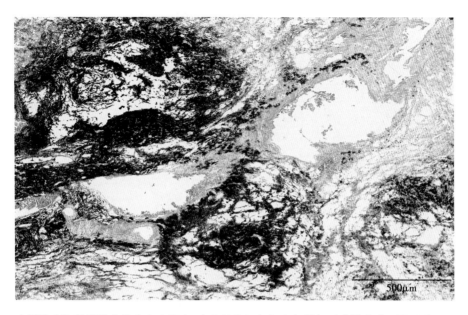

大量煤尘沉积似结节状分布在肺内，中心部位组织坏死与崩解形成煤尘池。周围肺组织弥漫性间质纤维化。（H.E 染色）
Abundant coal dust deposits in a nodular pattern, and the central coal dust deposits, admixed with tissue debris, may develop to "coal dust pool". Note a peripheral accumulation of collagen fibers. (H.E stain)

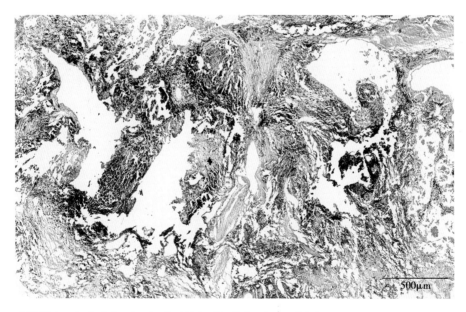

大量煤尘沉积在肺内，肺组织弥漫性间质纤维化。（H.E 染色）
Microscopic view of lung shows abundant coal dust deposits, accompanied by diffuse interstitial fibrosis. (H.E stain)

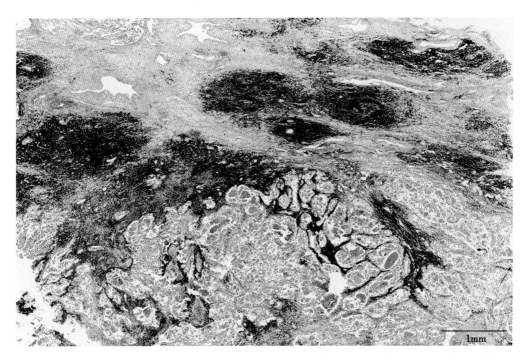

较多的煤尘沉积在肺内胸膜侧,形成胸膜下煤尘细胞灶和煤尘纤维灶,肺内可见浸润性生长的癌组织。(H.E 染色)

Multiple coal dust deposits in the subpleural tissue, creating cellular coal dust foci and fibrous coal dust foci. Cancer cells are infiltrated in the lung. (H.E stain)

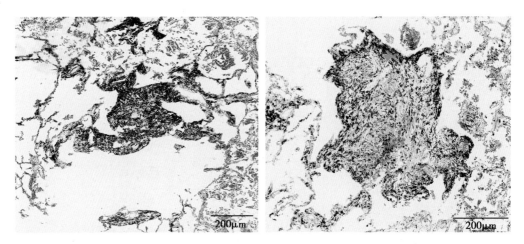

左图显示煤尘沉积在肺内形成煤尘细胞灶伴灶周肺气肿。右图显示肺内非典型煤矽结节形成。(H.E 染色)

Left photography illustration of cellular coal dust foci surrounded by emphysema. Right one evidence of atypical coal silicotic nodule in lung. (H.E stain)

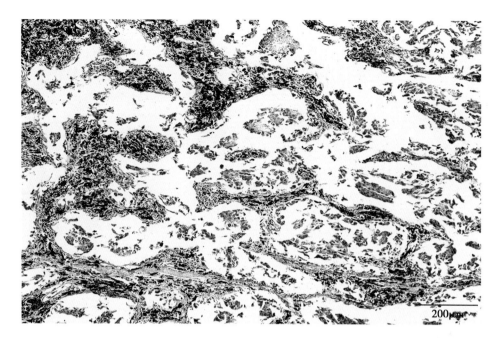

较多煤尘沉积在肺间质。癌组织呈小腺泡样、微乳头样结构在肺泡腔内浸润性生长。(H.E 染色)

Microscopic view of adenocarcinoma illustrates the invasion of airspace by glands or micropapillae of tumor cells. Note pulmonary interstitial tissue with multiple coal dust deposits. (H.E stain)

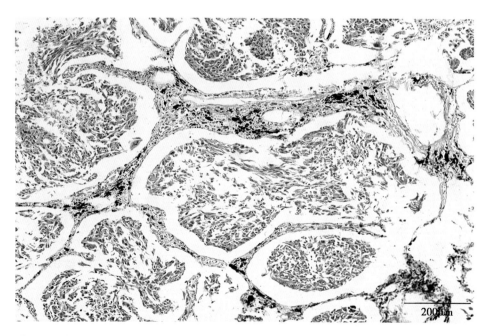

煤尘沉积在肺间质。癌组织充填在肺泡腔内。(H.E 染色)

High power view shows the alveolar spaces packed with cancer cells and alveolar septum deposited by coal dust. (H.E stain)

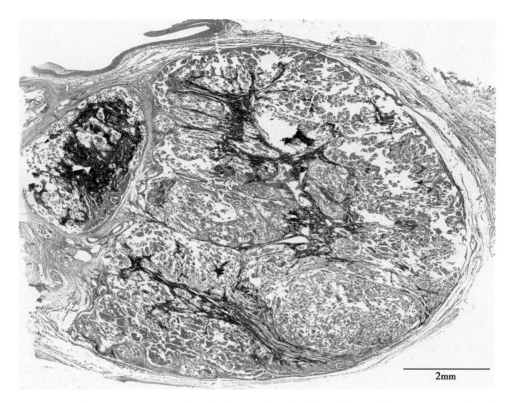

2mm

肺门淋巴结内腺癌组织弥漫浸润性生长破坏淋巴结原有结构,其间可见较多煤尘的沉积伴间质纤维化。(H.E 染色)
Schematic illustration of coal dust deposition and interstitial fibrosis in lymph nodes, with normal tissue destruction by adenocarcinoma cells. (H.E stain)

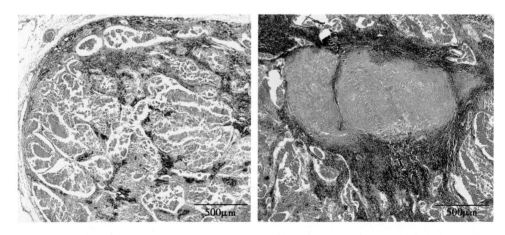

500μm   500μm

左图显示肺腺癌淋巴结内的转移;右图显示肺腺癌转移的淋巴结内煤矽结节的形成。(H.E 染色)
Left photography shows lymph node adenocarcinoma metastasis; while the right one reveals coal silicotic nodules in the lymph node with adenocarcinoma metastasis. (H.E stain)

案例七

煤肺Ⅰ期(煤斑－气肿)合并肺源性心脏

职业史

男性,54岁,井下采煤工作18年,通风1年。

临床情况

慢性支气管炎、肺气肿病史10余年,日渐加重。于1978年先后多次住院治疗,于1985年12月5日病情加重治疗无效死亡。

临床体检:桶状胸,肋间隙增宽,叩诊过清音,双肺可闻及干鸣音。肝脏边界在剑突下4cm。

心电图:窦性心动过速,心电轴右偏,肺型P波,完全性右束支传导阻滞。

X线胸片:双肺透过度增加,细网状纹理。可见小结节状阴影。

入院诊断为慢性支气管炎,肺气肿,肺心病伴心衰。心源性肝硬化,腹水,肾功能衰竭。

尸检情况

大体检查:①两肺:表面可见的黑色煤斑灶,遍布全肺并相互融合,以两肺上叶及脊柱侧为重。左肺肺尖处可见数个大泡型肺气肿形成。右肺肺尖处可见2个栗子大小的肺大疱。左肺上叶外侧中下3/4范围内有广泛的纤维性粘连,胸膜明显增厚。双肺叶间裂有广泛的纤维性粘连(见图谱中图5右图)。②心脏:体积增大,重量增加(350g),心尖圆顿,为扩大的右心室构成。左心室转向至左下后方。右心房5cm×5cm,右心室肥大,部分肉柱、乳头肌增粗,室上嵴突出于心内膜面(约5.5cm×2.5cm),肺动脉瓣下2cm处右室壁厚度达6mm(见图谱中图44)。左心室壁厚1.2cm,左心室腔无明显扩张。

显微镜检查:①两肺:可见煤尘沉积在肺内小血管、呼吸性细支气管、小叶间隔及胸膜下,形成诸多煤斑、煤尘细胞灶和煤尘纤维灶,伴小叶中心型肺气肿,肺内弥漫性肺间质纤维化。肺泡壁小血管扩张、充血及出血。局部肺泡腔内可见浆液性渗出物、炎细胞渗出及红细胞的漏出。局部肺泡壁Ⅱ型上皮细胞增生。肺内小动脉管壁增厚、中层平滑肌细胞增生。②心脏:右心室心肌纤维增粗,核大、深染,呈不规则形。右室心肌组织可见局灶状坏死、部分病变的心肌组织被纤维化的纤维组织取代(灶状瘢痕形成)。心肌间质水肿和纤维组织增生。

病理诊断:煤肺 I 期

1. 肺内煤斑灶,伴小叶中心性肺气肿接近肺容积 50%。肺内间质纤维化接近 1 级 /1 度。

2. 肺门、气管叉、气管旁、穷隆下淋巴结内煤尘沉积及纤维组织增生。

3. 慢性支气管炎、肺气肿、肺大泡形成。

4. 右心室肥大(右室壁厚 6mm),肺内小动脉肌层增厚。

5. 主动脉、肺动脉主干粥样硬化。冠状动脉(前降支、左旋支)粥样硬化。

Case 7

Anthracosis
(stage I, Coal dust maculae and emphysema) with cor pulmonale

Age: 54 years

Sex: Male

Occupational History:

The patient had been performed coal mining and ventilation work for 18 years and 1 year respectively.

Medical History:

More than ten years of chronic bronchitis and emphysema, and clinical treatment could not ameliorate the patient's symptoms since 1978. On December 5, 1985, after the rescue battlement, he unfortunately died.

When he was in hospital, physical examination found barrel chest and widened intercostals space, hyperresonance and wheezes, enlarged liver whose lower margin reaches at the level of 4cm below the xiphoid process. Electrocardiogram showed abnormal results, including sinus tachycardia, right deviation of electrocrdiac axis, pulmonary P wave, and complete right bundle branch block. X-ray revealed an increased lucent lung with increased lung marking and micronodular shadows. Therefore, his diagnosis included chronic bronchitis and emphysema, cor pulmonale with heart failure, cardiogenic liver cirrhosis with ascites, and renal failure.

Autopsy examination of the lung and the heart:

Gross: ①Lung: The black maculae are diffusely distributed in lungs, and more severe in the upper lobes or close to the spine. The tips of lungs illustrate bullous emphysema, evidenced by several small bullae in the left lung and two bullae, as large as chestnut, in the right lung. In the upper lobe of the left lung with thickened pleura, extensive area of fibrous adhesion occurs in the lower and middle third of lateral, do the same close to the interlobar fissure of lungs (the right photography of Fig.5). ②Heart: The heart has increased mass and weight (350g), with blunt apex composed by the enlarged right ventricle. The left ventricle shifts to the posterior lower left of the heart, with a, 1.2cm in thickness, wall and normal lumen. The area of right atria reaches at 5.0cm*5.0cm, accompanied with right ventricular hypertrophy, showing the thickening partial trabeculae carneae and papillary muscle, supraventricular crest poking up above the endothelium, maximal thickness of right ventricle wall being 6mm (location is at the level of 2cm below pulmonary valve) (Fig.44).

Histology: ①Lungs: Abundant coal dust deposits around the small blood vessels, respiratory bronchioles, interlobular septum or under the pleura, producing multiple coal dust dots, cellular coal dust foci and fibrous coal dust foci, with centrilobular emphysema and diffuse interstitial fibrosis. The congested septal capillaries, inflammatory cells exudation and erythrocyte transudation correspond to inflammation response. In addition, type II epithelial cells hyperplasia, small arteries wall thickening with proliferated smooth muscle cells are visible in lung. ②Heart: Microscopically, myocyte diameter increases, associated with prominent irregular nuclear enlargement. The patchy areas of necrotic tissue occur in the right ventricle, some of which are replaced by dense collagenous scar, with edema and fibrous proliferation in the interstitial tissue.

Pathological Diagnosis:

1. Anthracosis (stage I): It is supported by coal dust maculae surrounded by centrilobular emphysema (nearly 50% of the pulmonary volume), accompanied with interstitial fibrosis (grade I).

2. Coal dust deposition and fibrous proliferation in the lymph nodes of hilum, bifurcation of tracheas, para tracheas, subfornix.

3. Chronic bronchitis and emphysema with bullae formation.

4. Right ventricular hypertrophy (6mm of right ventricular wall thickness), with thickened muscularis of small arteries.

5. Atherosclerosis of aorta, pulmonary artery, coronary artery (anterior descending branch, left circumflex branch).

案例七 附图（Appendix of case 7）

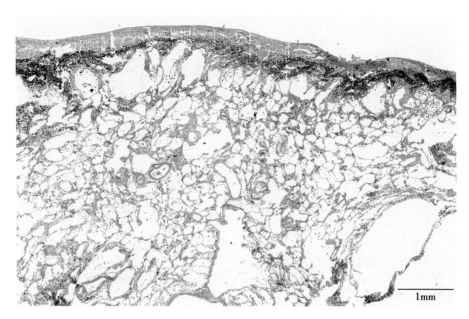

大量煤尘沉积在胸膜伴纤维组织增生，胸膜显著增厚。胸膜下方肺组织内小气道与肺泡腔扩张。（H.E 染色）

Abundant coal dust, admixed with proliferated fibrous tissue, thicken the pleura obviously, with subpleural emphysema characterized by small airway and airspaces enlargement. (H.E stain)

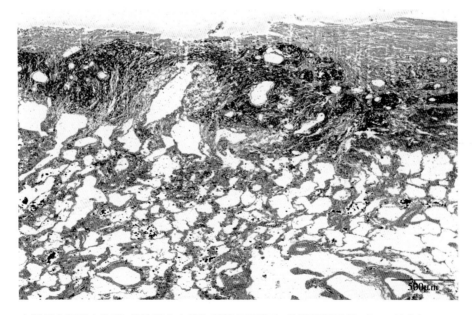

大量煤尘沉积在胸膜，伴胸膜小血管和纤维组织增生，胸膜显著增厚。（H.E 染色）

The thickened pleura contain multiple coal dust deposits, proliferated fibrous tissue and small blood vessels. (H.E stain)

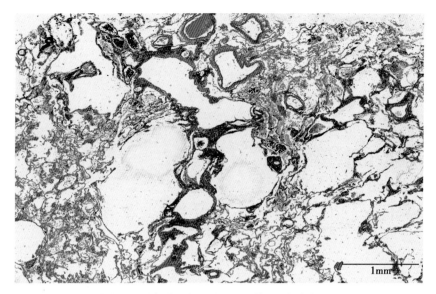

较多煤尘沉积在肺内细小支气管、肺泡壁及小血管壁,伴肺内小动脉壁增厚及小叶中心型肺气肿形成。(H.E 染色)

Morderate coal dust deposits around small bronchi, bronchioles, alveolar septum and thickened small blood vessels wall, with interlobular emphysema. (H.E stain)

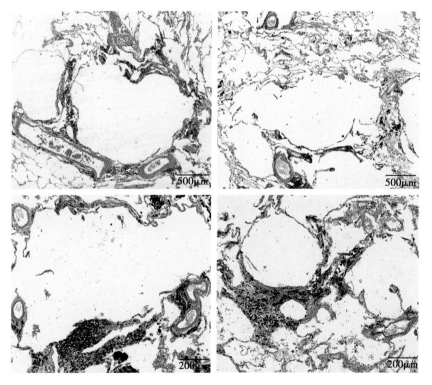

煤工尘肺伴肺气肿形成。(H.E 染色)

Coal works' pneumoconiosis with emphysema. (H.E stain)

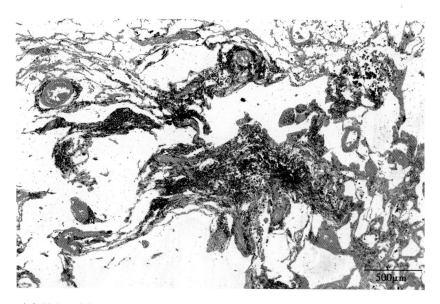

肺内煤尘细胞灶和煤尘纤维灶形成。细小支气管壁与肺泡壁可见较多扩张充血的小血管，血管壁增厚。（H.E 染色）

Microscopic view of lung illustration of cellular coal dust foci and fibrous coal dust foci. Note the congested thickened small blood vessels in the wall of small bronchi, bronchioles, and alveolar septum. (H.E stain)

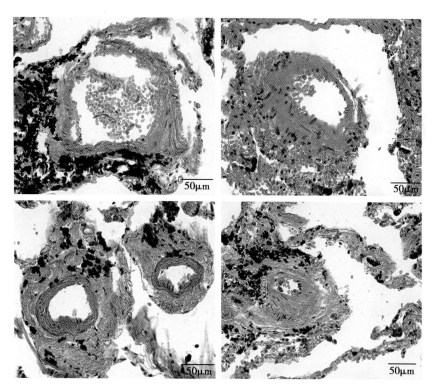

煤工尘肺伴肺内小血管增生。肺内小动脉平滑肌层增生、管壁增厚。（H.E 染色）

Coal works' pneumoconiosis with proliferated small blood arteries. Smooth muscle cells proliferation causes thickening of small artery wall. (H.E stain)

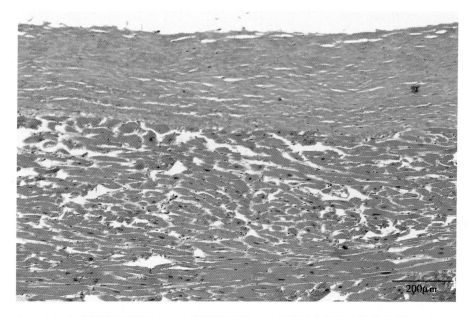

右心室心内膜纤维组织增生，心内膜明显增厚。心内膜下方部分心肌细胞肥大。(H.E 染色)

High power view of heart illustration of the thickening endocardium with proliferated fibrous tissue and patchy areas of myocyte hypertrophy under the endocardium. (H.E stain)

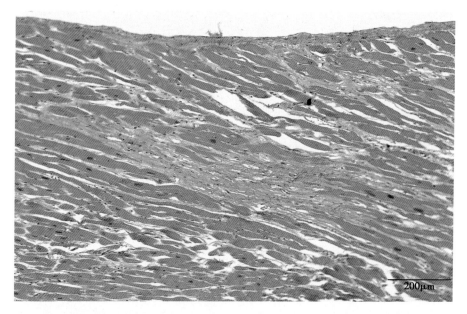

右心室心内膜下方部分心肌组织被增生的纤维组织取代（心肌瘢痕）。瘢痕灶周边部分心肌细胞肥大。(H.E 染色)

Microscopic photography shows the replacement of myocyte by proliferated collagenous fibers under the endocardium of right ventricle, with the surrounding myocyte hypertrophy. (H.E stain)

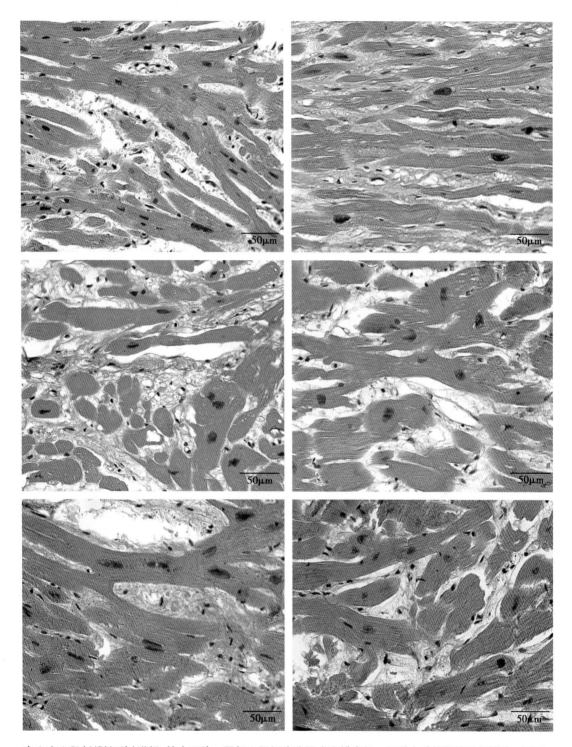

右心室心肌纤维(细胞)增粗,核大深染。局部心肌细胞分叉或交错走行。间质水肿伴纤维组织增生。(H.E
染色)

Myocyte diameter of right ventricle is increased, associated with deeply blue nuclear enlargement. A patchy area of myocyte in a interlacing pattern is seen, with edema and fibrous proliferation in the interstitial tissue. (H.E stain)

后 记

《煤工尘肺病理学图谱》一书,在编著者们共同努力下,顺利完成。该书是以内蒙古、山西、湖南、河北等省、自治区的煤矿井下工人尸检标本为材料,通过对大体和显微镜下尘肺病变的观察,力图展示煤矿工人尘肺病变复杂、形态多样的特点。特别是结合免疫组化和一些特殊染色,揭示了尘肺纤维化病变某些病理变化的特征。为深入了解煤工尘肺发病机制及其形态学的变化规律,提供一些有益的理论与临床信息。

在整理《煤工尘肺病理学图谱》一书的原始尸检病例与材料时,我们感慨万分。华北理工大学(原华北煤炭医学院)病理学系的许多同仁们为此书材料的获取、整理与珍藏付出过巨大的努力,留下了这些弥足珍贵的史料。

在这里我们首先要向李铁生、李洪珍两位前辈致敬!是他们开启了煤矿工人尘肺病理研究的先河,引领我们在尘肺研究领域不断探索、前行。他们编著的《煤矿尘肺病理组织学图谱》是一部经典的教科书,更是我们这本书著的"灵魂"。

感谢曾参加过尸检与诊断的老师、同仁们,他们有:张素华、王献华、佟树文、张小萍、刘京跃、郑素琴、李琪佳!

感谢李铁生、李万德、张尚明、王献华、郑素琴、孙影几任教研室(系)领导,对史料的惠存与保护!

感谢马文东、户万秘、向聚才、张玉强、荣玲等技术人员对大体与切片标本的制作!

感谢李倩、刘岩两位年轻人,协助拍摄与扫描大体与切片标本!

感谢参与标本制作、特殊染色、材料补充的博士与硕士研究生们!

感谢病理学系所有教职员工在前往新校区搬迁过程中对标本与尸检史料的爱护!

感谢张祥宏教授对此书病理形态学诊断方面的指导与帮助!

感谢赵金桓教授给予此书的支持与帮助!

感谢国家自然科学基金项目(81972988、81673119、81472953、81302395、81202162、81072254)的资助与支持!

向曾为此书付出过努力与做出贡献的各位同仁们一并致以诚挚的谢意!

编　者
2020 年 9 月

Acknowledgement

With the joint effort of contributors, the book Pathology Atlas of Coal Worker's Pneumoconiosis was successfully completed. With the autopsy specimens of underground coal workers in Inner Mongolia, Shanxi, Hunan, Hebei, and other provinces and autonomous regions, through the observation of the gross specimen and the pathological changes under the microscope, the book tries to demonstrate the complexity and diversity of coal worker's pneumoconiosis. Especially, through the combination of immunohistochemistry and some special stainings, this book unveils the characteristics of some pathological changes of pneumoconiosis fibrosis. It provides valuable theories and clinical information to the deep understanding of the pathogenesis of coal worker's pneumoconiosis and its morphological changes.

When we sorted out the original autopsy cases and materials for the book Pathology Atlas of Coal Worker's Pneumoconiosis, so many feelings came to our mind. Colleagues of the Department of Pathology of North China University of Science and Technology (previously known as North China Coal Medical College) have made great efforts to acquire, sort out, and preserve the materials for this book, leaving these precious historical materials.

We hereby paid our respects to Tiesheng Li and Hongzhen Li first! It is you who started the pathological study of coal worker's pneumoconiosis and lead us to constantly explore and move forward in this field. Pathology Atlas of Coal Mine Pneumoconiosis is a classical textbook, and is also the 'soul' of our book.

We want to express our gratitude to teachers and colleagues who have participated in the autopsy and diagnosis, including Suhua Zhang, Xianhua Wang, Shuwen Tong, Xiaoping Zhang, Jingyue Liu, Suqin Zheng, Qijia Li.

We want to express our gratitude to Tiesheng Li, Wande Li, Shangming Zhang, Xianhua Wang, Suqin Zheng, Ying Sun who were once leaders of the teaching and research office (department) for the preservation and protection of the historical materials!

We want to express our gratitude to Wendong Ma, Wanmi Hu, Jucai Xiang, Yuqiang Zhang, Ling Rong, and other technicians for making the gross and section specimens!

We want to thank the two youngsters Qian Li and Yan Liu for their assistance in the photographing and scanning of gross and section specimens!

We want to thank doctor and master students for their participation in specimen making, special staining, and the supplement of materials!

We want to thank the faculty of the Department of Pathology for their care when specimens and historical materials of autopsy were moved to the new campus!

We want to thank Professor Xianghong Zhang for his instructions and assistance with respect to the pathological and morphological diagnosis in this book!

We want to thank Professor Jinhuan Zhao for his support and help!

We want to thank the National Natural Science Foundation of China (No. 81972988、81673119、81472953、81302395、81202162、81072254) for the support on this work!

We hereby express our sincerest gratitude to all the colleagues who have made efforts and contributions to this book!

Authors
September, 2020